AN

ENQUIRY

INTO THE

STATISTICS AND PATHOLOGY

OF

SOME POINTS CONNECTED

WITH

ABSCESS IN THE LIVER,

AS MET WITH IN THE EAST INDIES

AN ENQUIRY

INTO THE

STATISTICS AND PATHOLOGY

OF

SOME POINTS CONNECTED

WITH

ABSCESS IN THE LIVER,

AS MET WITH IN THE EAST INDIES

BY

EDWARD JOHN WARING

GYAN

Published by

Gyan Publishing House
5, Ansari Road
Daryaganj, New Delhi-110002
Phone: 011-47034999, 9811692060
E-mail: books@gyanbooks.com

Distribution Network
gyanbooks.com
India, USA, Canada, UK, Australia, France

ISBN: 978-93-6280-085-5 (PB)

First Published, 1854

2nd Impression 2023

Printed at: Gyan Press, Delhi.

AN ENQUIRY INTO THE STATISTICS AND PATHOLOGY OF SOME POINTS CONNECTED WITH ABSCESS IN THE LIVER, AS MET WITH IN THE EAST INDIES
Author: EDWARD JOHN WARING

AN ENQUIRY INTO THE STATISTICS AND PATHOLOGY OF SOME POINTS CONNECTED WITH ABSCESS IN THE LIVER, AS MET WITH IN THE EAST INDIES,

BY

EDWARD JOHN WARING,

RESIDENCY SURGEON AT TRAVANCORE.

Trevandrum:

GOVERNMENT PRESS—W. WELLS, PRINTER.

1854.

TO

LIEUTENANT-GENERAL W. CULLEN,

MADRAS ARTILLERY,

BRITISH RESIDENT AT TRAVANCORE AND COCHIN,

THIS TREATISE IS RESPECTFULLY DEDICATED,

AS A SMALL MARK OF

SINCERE PERSONAL ESTEEM,

BY HIS OBLIGED AND VERY OBEDIENT SERVANT,

EDWARD J. WARING.

PREFACE.

In conducting the following investigation, I have acted throughout in the character of a learner, an enquirer, a searcher after truth; I have had no theories to support, no foregone conclusions to substantiate.

The history of the following paper, and the circumstances which led to its compilation, are simply these. On first joining the Indian Medical Service, two most highly interesting cases of hepatic abscess fell under my observation in the Artillery Hospital at St. Thomas's Mount, under the charge of my friend, Dr. George Pearse. I contrasted, in no complimentary manner as far I was concerned, his intimate and thorough knowledge of the disease he was treating, with my own ignorance of its history and pathology; and I resolved to allow no opportunity to pass, without making myself acquainted with it. I, accordingly, made notes of all such cases as fell under my observation in the course of my reading, and the notes thus collected, I now venture to put into print, feeling convinced that to a large number of young medical officers in India, they will prove an acceptable addition to our present stock of information on Indian diseases. To some of the senior members of the service, I also venture to hope that this investigation will be neither uninteresting nor unacceptable.

The present enquiry is strictly limited to hepatic abscess as it occurs in the East Indies; and it will be seen that all the collected cases commenced, progressed, and terminated, (whether in death or in recovery,) in some portion of our Indian Possessions. This restriction was found necessary, in order to obviate many objections which might otherwise have been raised to the conclusions attempted to be drawn: the strength which would have been gained by a few additional numbers, would have been more than counter-balanced by the objections which might reasonably have been raised as to the influence of climate, the different class of persons affected, the comparatively unimpaired condition of the constitution in persons inhabiting a cold or temperate clime, &c., had cases occurring in England and other extra-tropical countries been included in the list.

From various sources, I have collected 300 cases of hepatic abscess which terminated fatally, 81 in which the contents of the abscess were evacuated by operation, (many of these are included amongst the fatal cases,) and 25 in which spontaneous recovery took place. It has been found advisable to divide these into classes according to their respective terminations; and after a short detailed summary of the cases in each class, some deductions have been drawn, and such observations offered, as appeared to have an important bearing on the history and pathology of the disease under consideration.

I much regret that in the arrangement of the fatal cases, considerable irregularity will be found to exist; this has arisen from three causes. 1st. In the list I originally compiled, all cases, whether terminating in recovery or in death, and also all those in which the abscess was punctured, were placed together; and at the same time they were carefully tabulated according to symptoms, and post mortem appearances; subsequently, I found, that for the purpose of elucidating facts, it would be far preferable to place each class by itself: this was accordingly done, and the vacancies caused by this arrangement, were filled up by the cases which came the last in the list; this was done in order to prevent the necessity of re-tabulating the whole number, which would have involved an immense amount of labour, and have taken up more time than I could afford to dedicate to it. 2ndly. In the list I first made, I confined myself solely to such cases as had something like a complete history attached to them; and consequently, I omitted several, simply because no post mortem was given; whilst, on the other hand, I excluded some very important post mortems in which abscess in the liver was found, because they were attended by no previous history. This I found to be a great error, and I subsequently added several of these, feeling convinced that in an investigation like the present, no one well authenticated fact can be regarded as unimportant, or can be omitted without prejudice to the subject under consideration. The third cause arose from my own negligence, having passed over by mistake some few cases which ought to have been included in my first list. It was impossible to put these in their proper places, without upsetting the whole of my tabular arrangement.

These irregularities, however, are of no real consequence; they have in no way interfered with the ultimate results and the deductions drawn: besides which, to each case is carefully appended the source from which it is derived, and the authority on which it is given.

To the works of Annesley, Twining, Conwell, Geddes, Macpherson, and Allan Webb, I am indebted for many highly important and valuable cases; but my especial thanks are due to Mr. Samuel Rogers and Dr. Alexander Lorimer, the able editors of the six volumes of the Madras Quarterly Medical Journal, and also to many writers in the Transactions of the Medical and Physical Society of Bombay, particularly to Dr. Morehead and Messrs. Stovell and Leith.

Trevandrum,

September 1*st*, 1854.

CONTENTS.

SUMMARY

OF

THREE HUNDRED CASES

OF

FATAL HEPATIC ABSCESS.

No. 1.—T. McLean; æt. 33, in India 6 years, of spare habit; admitted November 13th, 1833, with dysentery, of which he had suffered a slight attack in the previous October. The symptoms of dysentery were well marked; in addition to these, he had pain in the left hypochondrium extending to the top and back of the *left* shoulder, increased on deep inspiration and pressure. He was bled, took calomel, ipecacuan, &c. This pain subsequently extended to the right side, and to the scrobiculus cordis—he had nausea and vomiting, but no rigors—stools, thin and bilious, latterly of nearly a natural colour, passed with little straining, and before death involuntarily. Blood drawn from the arm, was cupped and buffed. Pulse small and frequent, afterwards full and firm—tongue white—debility—restlessness—skin covered with cold damp perspiration four days before death on the 29th Instant.

Autopsy.—Liver enlarged, extending over the left hypochondrium—left lobe enlarged and converted into one mass of abscess, adhering to the diaphragm and the stomach. The abscess had almost penetrated through the coat of the latter—spleen enlarged—intestines blushed throughout—much contraction—colon and rectum extensively ulcerated—other viscera healthy—serous effusion in the thoracic cavity, and also in the brain. Heart healthy. (*Dr. J. Hutchinson, Madras Med. Journal,* vol. i, *p.* 120.)

No. 2.—T. Haywood, 8 years in India, a slender made man, of delicate appearance; admitted with hepatitis, July 29th; died August 29th. Symptoms and treatment not given.

Autopsy.—Left lobe of the liver very large, converted into one large abscess containing ten pints of pus. Two smaller abscesses were found in the right lobe, and numerous adhesions connected it to the stomach, large intestines, spleen and mesentery—condition of the intestines not given. (*Dr. F. Seivwright*, ibid, vol. i, *p.* 138.)

No. 3.—R. Platts, æt. 25, admitted Nov. 25th, 1835, with severe pain in the region of the liver, affecting his breathing and extending to the right shoulder—had been ill for 15 days—pulse quick and contracted, tongue loaded, urine scanty and high coloured, great thirst. He was bled, and took mercury till there was salivary discharge. Dec. 6th, salivary flow ceased, side and shoulder again uneasy, and the stools of a watery brown appearance. Dec. 12th, easier generally, skin cool, mouth again tender. He, however, gradually became worse; pain increased by pressure, no sleep, great prostration and dyspnæa. He died Dec. 19th.

Autopsy.—Liver an enormous mass of disease, strongly adhering to the diaphragm, and filling the left hypochondrium—one abscess in the centre of the right lobe contained 1 pound of pus; and there were three other abscesses protruding into the thoracic cavity, and adhering to the ribs. The large intestines throughout partially ulcerated. (*Dr. F. Seivwright*, ibid, *p.* 138.)

No. 4.—L. Page, æt. 30, of robust habit, a hard liver, admitted Dec. 12th, 1835, after a fit of intemperance, with pain in the right side, and he stated that he had been suffering with pain, fever, and nausea for the three previous days. He was depleted locally and generally, and took calomel until well marked ptyalism came on; this occurred four days before death. He had severe pain in the posterior region of the liver, which was much increased by the motion of a dooly, he being at the time on the line of march. He became greatly emaciated, and had much purging and prostration of strength. He died on the 29th.

Autopsy.—Liver twice its natural size, and rising high into the thorax; one abscess therein, the size of an orange, and several others dispersed through its substance. The large intestines ulcerated, and the mucous membrane in several places in a state of gangrene. (*Dr. F. Seivwright*, ibid, *p.* 139.)

No. 5.—Murphy, æt. 32, a large made man, admitted Dec. 8th, 1837, after some unusual exertion, with symptoms of pneumonia, which gradually gave way under treatment. It is not stated that he took any mercury. He was afterwards attacked with dysentery, and then with symptoms of hepatitis; but the signs of the latter so treacherously crept upon him, that it was only by watching, cross-questioning, and the aid of repeated examination under pressure with the hand, that it was confirmed—leeches, blisters, a seton, and alteratives, were employed, and though mercury was used internally and by friction, ptyalism could not be induced.

slight swelling of the gums, and a very slight taint of the breath, being all that could be detected. On February 1st, purging came on, and he died on the 14th.

Autopsy.—In the concave surface of the liver, about its centre anteriorly, was an abscess about the size of a billiard ball, containing a reddish brown and very fetid fluid, similar to that which had for some days been passed by stool. The walls of this cavity were of a dark livid colour, and of gangrenous odour. Gangrene had attacked the liver to a considerable depth; the gall bladder was no where to be seen, and appeared to have been completely disorganized. The abscess had become attached to the arch of the colon, on opening which a distinct perforation was seen, the lips of the aperture were red and inflamed; through this passage the contents of the abscess had been discharged into the colon, which was distended with dark gangrenous fluid, even up to the caput cæcum; its coats were somewhat thickened, but there was no ulceration. (*Dr. F. Seivwright*, ibid, vol. i, *p.* 147.)

No. 6.—R. Parke, æt. 34, admitted Feb. 6th, 1839, with severe pain over the whole of the right hypochondrium, augmented by pressure or deep inspiration—bowels relaxed—stools blackish—had been ill for 4 days, and had been attacked twice previously with hepatitis. He was depleted, and took calomel until ptyalism appeared. The pain in the liver abated, and he had no uneasiness in the hepatic region, except when he turned on the left side. The stools became of a reddish-yellow colour—he had also profuse sweats at night, debility and great emaciation, hiccup, œdema of the lower extremities, no pain in the shoulder, no rigors. The abscess was opened previous to death, March 14th. Case ii, in List of Operations.

Autopsy.—One immense abscess was found in the convex part of the right lobe of the liver, containing a few ounces of curdled matter. The colon was contracted in many parts, and there were cicatrices of former ulceration in the caput cæcum, sigmoid flexure, and rectum. The lower lobes of both lungs were highly congested and hepatized, and the right lung was adherent to the diaphragm. (*Dr. Murray*, ibid, vol. i, *p.* 473.)

No. 7.—Lieut. Bligh, H. M. 39th Regt., long subject to chronic bowel complaint: was admitted Feb. 6th, 1839, with chronic hepatitis.—Symptoms, a dragging pain in the right side, hectic fever with exhausting perspirations, nausea, vomiting, and cough with expectoration. The expectoration was slight, but by degrees nearly a pint of bloody puriform sputa came away in the 24 hours. On the 17th, the presence of bile was discovered in the sputa. There was no respiratory murmur below the mamma. Feet œdematous—delirium supervened—fluctuation being discovered, the abscess was opened on the 16th of March. All the symptoms much improved after the operation, but he remained very weak. The day before death (March 22nd) he passed by stool some red coloured matter, like that which came off from the abscess. He died in a fit of exhaustion.

Autopsy.—One large abscess, eight inches in diameter, existed in the right lobe of the liver; it communicated freely with the right lung, and its walls in the substance of the lung were strengthened by a distinct red layer of lymph. At the upper part of the cavity, the substance of the lung was quite soft and disorganized, and contained several vomicæ. The bronchial tubes opened into the softened mass by abrupt eroded orifices, thus pointing out the road through which the red sputa and pus had been expectorated. There was not merely one distinct opening, but all the inferior ramifications had the same kind of abrupt termination. The liver was very large, but without adhesions to the stomach or intestines. The hepatic tissue was livid, and inclined to green. On the anterior surface of the left lobe was a distinct cicatrix, but the subjacent tissue gave no evidence of the existence of abscess at any previous date. Case iii, in List of Operations. (*Dr. J. McGrigor*, ibid, vol. i, *p.* 476.)

No. 8.—J. Baker, æt. 37, admitted March 17th, 1840, and died June 17th, 1840—combined with dysentery—abscess opened 73 days before death—particulars not given. Case xl, in List of Operations.

Autopsy.—A large abscess occupied the whole of the left lobe of the liver, which had displaced the stomach, making its long diameter perpendicular instead of transverse. The abscess protruded into the chest; a very thin barrier, formed by the diaphragm, alone prevented its bursting into this cavity. The gall bladder contained a small quantity of orange coloured bile—colon ulcerated—some of the ulcers of old standing and healed, others in a state of ulceration. (*Register of H. M. 94th Regt., Madras Med. Journal*, vol. vi, *p.* 325.)

No. 9.—Stokes, æt. 30, dark complexion, melancholic temperament, temperate habits, admitted with dysenteric symptoms. Ptyalism was established, and the disease apparently subdued, but convalescence did not take place properly; his appetite did not return, his tongue continued foul, bowels irregular, and it was observed that the ptyalism had entirely subsided. Hepatic symptoms now appeared, there was a degree of tenderness in the region of the liver, increased slightly on drawing a full breath. There was no particular constitutional disturbance beyond want of appetite and indifferent rest; pulse 80, not excited; there was slight pain in the epigastrium. Amongst other remedies, calomel, to the extent of 210 grains was given, but it failed entirely to affect the mouth. He always lay with the greatest comfort on his left side, although he could lie on either side; tongue moist, but foul to the very tip. He died in January 1838.

Autopsy.—Liver much enlarged, firm, of a pale colour, utterly destitute of blood or bile, right lobe slightly adherent to the side; in it were three distinct abscesses, containing about lbiv of purulent matter; besides these there were several small abscesses, immediately under the peritoneal coat. The gall bladder, flaccid, of the colour of wash-leather, contained some pale straw coloured bile. Cæcum enlarged, and on its mucous coat were a few indolent ulcers; other viscera healthy. (*Dr. McDonnell*, ibid, vol. ii, *p.* 33.)

No. 10.—James, a young man of sanguine temperament, admitted with a third attack of dysentery. He had been several days in hospital, and actively treated before he began to feel pain in the side, and at first it was so diffused that he could not specify where it was. The pain was now referred to the top of the shoulder, and he lay constantly on the left side, the right side showing evident enlargement, and in the epigastrium was a fluctuating tumour. The bowels were at first irritable, the stools highly acrid and bilious, mixed with slime and blood, but latterly they much improved. The pulse was excited, with a jerk in it: the pain was latterly not complained of, the tongue became furred, quite to the tip; there were evening exacerbations, and gradual loss of strength, but no rigors. The two last days of his life, his breathing became attended with a mucous râle, and pus was expectorated. No mention is made of the administration of mercury.

Autopsy.—Liver much enlarged, particularly the left lobe, which was pale, firm, and gritty when incised. The right lobe, adherent to the diaphragm, contained four distinct abscesses; one under the epigastrium containing one ounce of good pus, a smaller one adjoining, and two deep seated; one of these had penetrated the diaphragm and communicated with the lung; the whole quantity of pus being about a quart, mesenteric glands enlarged. Extensive effusion of serum and lymph in the right thorax. (*Dr. McDonnell*, ibid, *p.* 36.)

No. 11.—A young man admitted with dysentery, upon which

hepatic symptoms supervened; there was a heavy pain in the side, which bulged out and was conspicuously enlarged, compared with the other side, which appeared quite flat; there was constant febrile excitement, aggravated in the evening; tongue brown and furred to the tip; the stools at first dysenteric, became feculent, and occasionally formed and natural. Hectic fever and profuse perspirations set in, and he died in December, 1838. The treatment consisted of local depletion, blue-pill, ipecacuanha, &c.

Autopsy.—The liver an immense size; the right lobe converted into an immense abscess, holding three quarts of pus. In the colon and cæcum were several small ulcers in a clean healing state. (*Dr. McDonnell,* ibid, *p.* 36.)

No. 12.—A seaman, æt. 39, 2 years in India, admitted with hepatic symptoms supervening on a bowel complaint. The symptoms yielded in a measure to treatment, but the mercury used, though it affected his mouth, did not produce healthy ptyalism, nor did he convalesce as he would have done, had the disease been overcome. The symptoms were obscure: there was indeed some fulness, extending from one hypochondrium to the other, but there was no particular spot, in which local examination afforded unequivocal evidence of the existence of matter. The abscess was opened, but with temporary benefit; he died two days after the operation.

Autopsy.—Liver much enlarged, occupying both hypochondria, the stomach being altogether concealed and pushed backwards by the left lobe. In the right lobe were three distinct abscesses; the contents of one of these, in the inferior portion of the lobe, appeared to be retained simply by the peritoneal covering of the viscus somewhat thickened, and adherent strongly to the contiguous viscera and the upper part of the right kidney. There was also an abscess in the left lobe. All these abscesses contained thick, healthy, purulent matter. Condition of the intestines not given. Case v, in List of Operations. (*Dr. W. Mortimer*, ibid, vol. ii, *p.* 225.)

No. 13.—J. Gorman, æt. 33, admitted February 8th, 1840, with fever, cough, dyspnæa, mucous expectoration, and daily rigors at noon. The principal subsequent symptoms were a frequent tickling cough, great difficulty of breathing, a sense of weight in the hepatic region, œdema of the body and legs, loss of appetite, great thirst, much prostration of strength, pulse 120 and intermitting. Decubitus on the left side or the back extremely oppressive, countenance anxious, hectic fever, and profuse night sweats. Although the liver was evidently enlarged, there was no fluctuation perceptible, it was slightly tender to the touch, and the right rectus muscle was more tense than the left; or, rather, it became so, on attempting to examine the liver. The urine sometimes contained a considerable puriform deposit, but latterly, after the abscess had been opened, it became clear. The bowels were "open" and "free," but without purging. He died March 18th, eleven days after the abscess had been punctured. The treatment previous to the operation, is not given; no mention is made of the administration of mercury.

Autopsy.—Liver much enlarged; the right lobe contained three large abscesses, one on the right side of the convex surface contained 1½ pint of thick, yellow, greenish pus. Immediately above this, was another empty contracted sac which had been punctured, and at the centre of the upper convex part of the liver was a third abscess, holding 3 pints of matter; this formed a prominent tumour, and pushed the diaphragm as high as the 4th rib. Gallbladder contracted and of a pale colour. In the thorax were about 5 pints of darkish serum. Case viii, in List of Operations. (*Dr. W. C. Maclean*, ibid, vol. ii, *p.* 232.)

No. 14.—Long in hospital, with occasional pains in the liver and shoulder, irregular bowels, frequency and stringiness of pulse, debility and gradual emaciation. Died in 1839. Treatment not given.

Autopsy.—A very large abscess was found occupying the right lobe of the liver. (*Dr. Geddes*, ibid, vol. ii, *p.* 311.)

No. 15.—Admitted with fever, June 6th, and died July 19th, 1839. There was very slight constitutional disturbance, from the second day after admission, till very nearly the period of his death. There was a slight yellow tinge in the eyes, countenance pale and unhealthy, urine red throughout. He had pain on pressure at the præcordia, and occasionally had "a stitch" in that locality. The bowels were at first constipated; on the 15th the bowels are reported as open, on the 25th regular. On the 28th, (22 days after admission with hepatic symptoms,) the bowels began to be irregular, and on the 12th of July, 7 days before death, they contained blood and mucous, but without griping or straining. The pulse stringy and irritable, never above 88 till the day before death. There was no fluctuation, and till very latterly no pain in the region of the liver, and then only very slight upon pressure. A sort of tympanitic puffing of the abdomen was noted on the 10th day. His mouth was made sore with mercury early in the disease—no rigors—he gradually sunk, and died July 19th.

Autopsy.—The edge of the right lobe extended down considerably beyond the ribs, was of a livid appearance, and contained lbij of yellow curdly matter of watery consistence. The intestines quite healthy. (*Dr. Geddes*, ibid, *p.* 312.)

No. 16.—J. Rose, æt. 41, 8 years in India, robust, healthy, active, of rather intemperate habits, admitted March 12th, 1838, with acute lancinating pain in the right iliac and hypochondriac regions, increased by pressure and motion, and accompanied by high fever, but without any dysenteric symptoms. Mercury was given early, but the system could not be brought under its influence. On the 15th, delirium tremens supervened; the pain ceased in a few days, but the fever remained, and was speedily followed by tympanitis, hectic sweats, and diarrhœa. He died April 8th. Fourteen days before admission he received a severe blow on the right side of the abdomen.

Autopsy.—The liver was firmly attached to the diaphragm, and contained the empty sac of a large abscess in the right lobe, which had discharged its contents into the right thoracic cavity, 20 ounces of bloody purulent matter being collected therein. The right lung was hepatized—gall bladder moderately filled with bile. Large intestines much inflated, but not ulcerated. The cæcum and ascending colon firmly adherent to the lumbar parietes and hollow of the os ilium; on separating this, a large abscess, containing 8 or 10 ounces of matter, was discovered, exterior to the gut, and extending from the kidney to the cavity of the pelvis. (*Dr. Shanks*, ibid, vol. iii, *p.* 17.)

No. 17.—J. Ross, æt. 53, 9 years in India, robust, corpulent, rather intemperate, admitted Aug. 8th, 1838, with acute pain in the side, vomiting and dysenteric purging, stools at first bloody and mucous, afterward shreddy and watery, and sanguineo—purulent, mixed occasionally with frothy, feculent evacuations; and followed by early prostration of strength, excessive irritability of stomach, cold, clammy sweats, and death on Sept. 2d. He was bled early in the disease, the blood being cupped and buffed, and calomel was given, at the same time that mercurial frictions were employed.

Autopsy.—Liver very large, with an immense abscess, holding 40 ounces of thick pus, in the posterior and inferior portion of the right lobe, the remainder of the liver, healthy. The large intestines, from the ileo-cæcal valve to the anus, were one mass of fleshy sloughing ulceration. The small intestines and other viscera healthy. (*Dr. Shanks*, ibid, vol. iii, *p.* 18.)

No. 18.—J. Sarsfield, æt. 28, temperate, well-conducted, admitted Sept. 21st, 1838, with a third relapse of dysentery, for which he had been actively treated. The last attack was apparently mild, and rather of a chronic character, but hectic and great prostration speedily followed, and he died, Nov. 10th. Throughout the whole of his illness he never complained of pain in the hepatic region, although latterly abscess was suspected. V. S. was employed, and he took calomel and opium in large doses.

Autopsy.—Liver much enlarged; in the centre of the left lobe, was an extensive abscess, containing 16 ounces of pus. The colon was distended, and its coats thickened; and on laying the intestine open, were found several patches of ulceration, in the cæcum, colon, and rectum, apparently in the progress of healing. In the arch of the colon were cicatrices of ulcers. The thoracic viscera healthy. (*Dr. Shanks*, ibid, vol. iii, *p.* 20.)

No. 19.—J. Varney, æt. 43, 9 years in India, a healthy, active man, of the most exemplary conduct and abstemious habits, admitted May 30th, 1839, with acute hepatitis, for which he was actively treated, and discharged apparently well, June 19th. Seven days after, (June 26th,) he was re-admitted with acute pain in the right side, vomiting, fever, and constipated bowels. He was bled, (blood cupped and buffed,) and amongst other things, took calomel in large doses, but without affecting his mouth. Abscess formed, accompanied with dysenteric stools, great prostration of strength, and profuse sweats. He died, July 12th, two days after the abscess had been opened.

Autopsy.—Liver much enlarged, adhering to the diaphragm and the ribs. Five abscesses, from the size of an orange to that of an egg, were found on the convex surface of the right lobe, and there were several others in the substance of both lobes. Throughout the whole of the mucous coat of the colon, were patches of incipient ulceration. The thoracic viscera healthy. Case xvi, in List of Operations. (*Dr. Shanks*, ibid, *p.* 32.)

No. 20.—H. Woods, æt. 38, 9 years in India, healthy, robust, admitted August 30th, 1839, with fever, and acute pain in the right hypochondrium, extending to the shoulder, increased by full inspiration and pressure—pulse 100, full and strong—skin hot and moist. The disease progressed rapidly; abscess opened on September 11th; he sunk on the following day. Blood drawn early in the case, was intensely buffed and cupped; mercury, though given in scruple doses, with mercurial friction, failed to affect the system.

Autopsy.—Liver enormous, weighing 8½ pounds, thrusting the diaphragm as high as the 4th rib. It was studded throughout with innumerable abscesses, from the size of a walnut to that of an orange; the entire substance was softened and disorganized. The colon was contracted, thickened, and closely studded throughout with granular ulceration. Case xvii, in List of Operations. (*Dr. Shanks*, ibid, *p.* 33.)

No. 21.—J. Randal, æt. 34, 9 years in India, well-conducted, had four previous attacks of hepatitis, but it is not stated, whether, amongst other remedies, mercury was administered. Admitted April 21st, 1839, with well marked symptoms of suppuration of the liver, consequent, apparently, upon an attack of hepatitis, six weeks before, for which he had been most actively treated. The abscess was opened, and the discharge was profuse for some weeks; diarrhœa, with cough and muco-purulent expectoration, then supervened, and he died June 21st.

Autopsy.—Adhesion between the liver and side. Innumerable small abscesses existed on the upper and under surfaces of the viscus, and also throughout its substance. The gall bladder was distended with thick, dark bile, like tar, the pancreas enlarged, the sigmoid flexure of the colon and rectum thickened and ulcerated. Case xv, in List of Operations. (*Dr. Shanks*, ibid, *p.* 33.)

No. 22.—J. Carroll, æt. 36, 9 years in India, a delicate looking man, discharged from hospital ten days previously, apparently quite recovered from a severe attack of dysentery and intermittent fever; was re-admitted Sept. 25th, 1839, with a relapse of dysentery, accompanied with tenderness on pressure over the colon. On October 3rd, he complained *for the first time,* of acute pain in the region of the liver, attended with fulness and hardness. The pain yielded to leeches and blisters, (mercury ?) but he continued pale and weakly, and had night sweats. Abscess evacuated Oct. 20th: he much improved for five weeks, when diarrhœa supervened, and he died Dec. 6th, 47 days after the operation.

Autopsy.—Liver adherent to the abdominal parietes, diaphragm and ribs; on separating these adhesions, the sac of an immense abscess was found, occupying the convex surface of the right lobe, penetrating nearly through the whole of its substance, which was quite disorganized, and converted into a mass of thick sloughy matter. The lower part of the abscess adhered to the arch of the colon, the mucous coat of which exhibited traces of former ulceration throughout its whole extent. Case xviii, in List of Operations. (*Dr. Shanks*, ibid, vol. iii, *p.* 34.)

No. 23.—T. Lancaster, æt. 38, 9 years in India, temperate, well-conducted. Within four months he had been twice in hospital, with dysentery and hepatitis, and on each occasion he had been actively treated; on the first occasion he was salivated. He was re-admitted with fatal attack January 8th, 1840, having been discharged, apparently well, only six weeks before. Counter-irritation, blue pill, and ipecacuanha, formed the main treatment. Died January 29th, three days after the abscess had been opened.

Autopsy.—Liver enlarged, adherent to the diaphragm and ribs. The whole of the right lobe was converted into the sac of an immense abscess, which had been punctured. There was general peritonitis, arising from the escape of matter (through the artificial opening) into the abdominal cavity. Case xix, in List of Operations. (*Dr. Shanks*, ibid, vol. iii, *p.* 35.)

No. 24.—W. McClare, æt. 33, 9 years in India, steady, well-conducted. He was in hospital, with apparently a mild attack of dysentery, from October 29th to November 16th; three days after his discharge he was re-admitted with a relapse, having painful distention of the abdomen, tenderness on pressure, great anxiety, restlessness, tormina and tenesmus, stools frequent and muco-sanguineous, alternating with healthy, feculent evacuations, followed by the discharge of a large cylindrical slough; great prostration, hiccup, and pain in the right side. He died 13 days after admission. Mercury made his mouth sore, but without ptyalism.

Autopsy.—Liver large, and thickly studded all over its upper and under surfaces, as well as throughout its substance, with small tubercles and abscesses of various sizes. The gall bladder moderately full of healthy looking bile. The caput cæcum and the ascending colon were much distended, and adhered firmly to the contiguous parietes, and on separating these adhesions, the coats were found to have sloughed, and given way in several places. (*Dr. Shanks*, ibid, vol. iii, *p.* 37.)

No. 25.—W. Holland, a delicate, strumous young man, often sick. The symptoms, which were very urgent, consisted principally of acute pain in the right hypochondrium, which extended in a lesser degree over the whole of the abdomen, tenderness on pressure, and retention of urine. Calomel was given in large doses, but without producing its specific effect on the system. He died on the 43d day of treatment.

Autopsy.—Liver enlarged, adherent to the ribs and diaphragm; the right lobe converted into a thin sac, which contained lbiii of thin, brownish coloured matter; gall bladder thickened and empty; cæcum pulpy and perforated, ascending colon in a state nearly approaching gangrene, right kidney enlarged, soft and bearing traces of recent inflammation. Serous effusion in the abdominal cavity—effusion of greenish serum (Oij) in the right side of the thorax, lungs tuberculated, heart flabby. (*Dr. Henderson,* ibid, vol. iii, *p.* 136.)

No. 26.—J. Madill, æt. 37, 6½ years in India, sickly, attenuated, frequently ill with hepatitis and dysentery, admitted March 27th, 1840, with nausea, fulness, and dull pain at the epigastrium and in the right hypochondrium, tongue coated, pulse weak and frequent, had diarrhœa for some days past. There was dull sound, over the hepatic region, on percussion, together with pain and fulness in the right iliac region. April 1st, "has occasional rigors, gums affected by mercury, frequent purging of watery fluid, tinged with blood,—is very low." Fluctuation becoming evident, the abscess was opened, and much matter evacuated; after this, he improved for a time, but he ultimately sunk, 97 days after the operation.

Autopsy.—Liver greatly enlarged, containing numerous large and deep seated abscesses, occupying its entire dimensions. The trocar had entered one situated at its lower edge; it contained much sanious pus, and seemed to communicate with the others. The colon ulcerated throughout. Case xxi, in List of Operations. (*Dr. Sinclair,* ibid, vol. iii, *p.* 187.)

No. 27.—J. Taylor, æt. 32, 4 months in India, stout, of swarthy complexion, was treated for pain in the side, without fever or any derangement of the general health: was discharged May 1st, and re-admitted a week afterwards with a return of pain in the right hypochondrium, no fulness of the side, nor rigors. Tongue, pulse, and skin, perfectly normal, bowels free. May 20th, "some fulness of the side apparent, but no fluctuation nor rigors. Mouth sore; a peculiar minute eruption over the face, arms, hands, and lower extremities; there is now much attendant fever." June 7th, "fulness continues, no rigors, nor pain on full inspiration." Fluctuation being perceptible, the abscess was opened; on the same evening, there was a sudden sinking of the powers of life, with pain over the abdomen, hiccup, &c. He died on the 9th, two days after the operation.

Autopsy.—Liver extensively disorganized, containing many large abscesses; one of these on the convex surface had been evacuated by puncture, and another on the concave surface had burst into the abdominal cavity, causing general inflammation and agglutination of the intestines. The bursting of this last abscess seems to have been the cause of this sudden sinking. Case xxii, in List of Operations. (*Dr. Sinclair,* ibid, vol. iii, *p.* 188.)

No. 28.—J. Lewsey, æt. 22, admitted May 30th, and died

September 23rd, 1840, ten days after the abscess had been opened, combined with dysentery. The symptoms and treatment not detailed.

Autopsy.—One abscess in the convex surface of the right lobe of the liver, (that punctured). Some small cicatrices of old ulcerations in the large intestines. Case xli, in List of Operations. (*Madras Medical Journal*, vol. vi, *p.* 326.)

No. 29.—W. Condy, æt. 19, admitted December 27th, and died April 26th, 1840, 87 days after the abscess had been opened. Symptoms and treatment not given.

Autopsy.—Liver small, light yellow buff colour, adherent to the side, on separating the adhesions a large abscess was found; there were also several small abscesses in the right lobe. Case xlii, in List of Operations. (*Ibid*, vol. vi, *p.* 326.)

No. 30.—H. McEvoy, æt. 35, 14 years in India, admitted April 28th, 1840, with feelings of general weakness, irritability of the stomach, and frequent vomiting. Bowels confined, pulse natural; had a previous attack of hepatitis. As the disease advanced, he had a dull heavy pain in the side, cold night sweats and cough, and he passed purulent matter both in his stools and urine. The liver was explored, as abscess was suspected, but no pus evacuated. He died June 17th, twenty days after the exploration. The treatment before the operation is not given.

Autopsy.—The right lobe of the liver adhered to the contiguous viscera, and contained two abscesses, one on the superior convex surface, communicating through the diaphragm with the right pleural cavity, and the inferior one had nearly penetrated the coats of the cæcum. The left lobe contained three small abscesses. (*Dr. Allman*, ibid, vol. iii, *p.* 194.)

No. 31.—J. Silver, æt. 37, 15 years in India, admitted August 1st, with acute pain in the right hypochondrium; this afterwards extended to the epigastrium, and in the latter position a swelling presented itself. He was languid, weak, and sallow, ptyalism occurred, but he remained restless at night, and had no appetite. The abscess was opened, after which he greatly improved for a time, but he ultimately sunk and died November 4th. Case xxv, in List of Operations.

Autopsy.—The right lobe of the liver was converted into the membraneous cyst of an abscess, containing upwards of 7 pints of purulent matter. There were strong adhesions to the side. (*Dr. Allman*, ibid, vol. iii, *p.* 194.)

No. 32.—F. Henwood, æt. 29, 12 years in India, admitted July 10th, 1840, with acute pain in the right hypochondrium, increased on pressure and on inspiration. In the subsequent course of the case, he had diarrhœa with tenesmus, and the stools contained purulent matter; he became much emaciated; there was hardness over the right lobe of the liver, tongue brown and coated, pulse 120. He died Aug. 5th, four days after the abscess had been opened. Case xxvi, in List of Operations.

Autopsy.—The liver adherent to the diaphragm and the side, no matter had escaped, but there were traces of inflammation on the peritoneum. The sac of the abscess was found adherent to and communicating with, the right kidney. The left lobe of the liver healthy. The right lung collapsed. It is to be regretted that amongst the symptoms the state of the urine is not mentioned. (*Dr. Allman,* ibid, vol. iii, *p.* 195.)

No. 33.—G. Veitch, æt. 38, sanguine temperament, admitted November 19th, 1814, with violent acute ophthalima, for which he was profusely bled and freely purged, at first every day; under this treatment the inflammation of the eyes subsided. On Nov. 28th, dysenteric symptoms came on, followed on December 1st, by acute hepatic symptoms. Mercury was used, externally and internally, but he got worse and died December 15th.

Autopsy.—The liver did not adhere to the diaphragm, and in the right lobe was an abscess which contained 29 oz. of white thick pus. Condition of the intestines not given. (*Dr. Nicoll,* ibid, vol. iii, *p.* 226.)

No. 34.—D. Jobson, æt. 21, admitted October 25th, 1841, died November 27th, the abscess having been opened the previous day. Symptoms and treatment not given. Case xliii, in List of Operations.

Autopsy.—Liver much enlarged, firmly adherent to contiguous parts, the substance studded throughout with numerous abscesses, which in some stage or another occupied the whole viscus. (*Register of H. M. 94th Regt.,* ibid, vol. vi, *p.* 326.)

No. 35.—J. Marshall, æt. 31, 7 years in India, stout, leucophlegmatic, was under treatment for dysentery from August 5th, to Sept. 5th, when he was discharged apparently well. Four days after, (Sept. 9th,) he was re-admitted with acute hepatitis; he was actively treated, and brought under the influence of mercury within three days after admission. His symptoms now nearly disappeared, but he never allowed that he was altogether free from pain about the left lobe of the liver, although his general health improved so much that he was permitted to walk about. On Sept. 30th, he was suddenly seized with weakness, approaching to fainting; this was instantly followed by severe aoute pain in the lower part of the left side of the abdomen, and a desire to go to stool; when removed from the night chair he was almost in a state of syncope. Evident symptoms of peritonitis now supervened, extreme tenderness over the abdomen increased by pressure, skin hot, pulse 100, sharp, urine scanty and high coloured. He was bled, had purgatives, &c., and on October 3rd, it is reported "there has been a gradual though slow amendment, the pain seems now to have entirely left the lower part of the abdomen, and is chiefly seated about the left lobe of the liver; he can now turn in bed with ease; (this formerly gave him great pain;) has scanty and mucous stools, pulse rather frequent, skin cool, thirst less." All progressed favourably till Oct. 12th, when he had another attack similar to the one on the 30th ultimo. Abdomen painful on pressure, pulse small and frequent, vomiting of bilious matter, clammy perspirations, great prostration of strength. He died on the 15th.

Autopsy.—A small abscess in the left lobe of the liver was found to have given way, and the matter escaped between the parietes of the abdomen and the intestines, until it reached the inside of the rim of the pelvis, where its further progress was arrested; the inflammation, which immediately took place, confined it in this position, so that when the body was examined, from 4 to 6 ounces of purulent matter were found, extending in a direct line of about four inches in breadth, from the opening in the liver to about Poupart's Ligament; this, and the natural effects of such a state, together with a slight enlargement of the liver, were the only morbid appearances observed on dissection. The abscess had evidently burst on Sept. 30th, 16 days before death. (*Dr. Henderson*, ibid, vol. iii, *p.* 332.)

No. 36.—J. McKenna, æt. 38, 7 years in India, an Irishman, delicate, intemperate, admitted Nov. 1st, 1832, with catarrhal fever. He was salivated by a small dose of calomel, and for this he was detained in hospital. The report on Nov. 18th is "for some days past he has had the appearance of falling off in his general health, but never allowed that there was any thing the matter with him until this morning; now he complains of having had a bad night, and also of pain in the right hypochondrium, increased on pressure; on examination there appears to be slight enlargement of the liver; cannot lie on the left side without greatly increasing the pain; pulse small, quick, but weak; skin rather below the usual temperature, thirst, loss of appetite, &c.; had one natural stool yesterday. This appears to be the first time he has been under treatment for hepatic disease." He slightly improved, but afterwards became worse, and died on the 25th, nine days after first complaining of his side. At no period does he appear to have had rigors, nor pain in the shoulder.

Autopsy.—In the liver was a large abscess, seemingly of some standing, containing two pints of thin matter. Mesenteric glands enlarged, right lung, small and indurated, and containing several small vomicæ. Spleen enlarged and soft, other viscera not diseased. (*Dr. Henderson,* ibid, *p.* 335.)

No. 37.—H. Shields, æt. 32, 5 years in India, Irish, very dissipated, admitted with hepatitis, and died March 31st, 1832. History of the case not given.

Autopsy.—The whole of the lower edge of the liver was connected to the peritoneum, lining the abdomen to the depth of 3 or 4 inches, forming a complete sac from the angle of the ribs on the right side, to the same point on the left; in this there was a considerable quantity of matter. The thin edge of the liver which was included in the sac had entirely disappeared, to the extent of about half an inch in depth. Liver enlarged and pale. (*Dr. Henderson,* ibid, *p.* 336.)

No. 38.—S. Peach, æt. 26, 6 years in India, delicate, admitted Sept. 1st, with remittent fever. Active measures were pursued, but afterwards hepatic disease became evident, the acute symptoms of which was relieved by the usual means (?) but the case terminated fatally in abscess, and he died Oct. 30th. Autopsy not given. (*Dr. Henderson,* ibid, *p.* 337.)

No. 39.—W. Wells, æt. 29, 8 years in India, stout habit, admitted with a second attack of dysentery, Aug. 9th, 1832. He was actively treated, and on the 27th, the report is "progressive amendment though slow, evacuations healthy, appetite good." On the 29th, symptoms of hepatitis set in, he was depleted and took calomel till his gums became tender; he then improved for a time, but ultimately died, Nov. 9th. For some time before death, a large quantity of purulent matter was thrown up from the lungs.

Autopsy.—The upper part of the right lobe of the liver was a complete mass of disease, in which the diaphragm and lungs were engaged; the diaphragm had given way, permitting the contents of a large abscess to escape into the right side of the thorax. (*Dr. Henderson,* ibid, *p.* 337.)

No. 40.—D. Hassen, æt. 33, 7 years in India, Irishman, admitted Nov. 12th, 1832, with dysentery—this was subdued but he continued weak, and at times complained of uneasiness in the colon, which he always ascribed to flatulence; his general health did not improve although he was able to take a little exercise, and he continued apparently free from his original complaint. On the

29th of Nov. he was suddenly seized with delirium; on the 30th he was again sensible, and stated that the only uneasiness he had was pain in the back of the right shoulder. The region of the liver was carefully and minutely examined the same evening; there was no increase of heat or fulness of the part, nor did he wince in the slightest degree under pressure; pulse and skin about their natural standard, tongue loaded and foul. During the remainder of the case, he complained of pain in the abdomen generally, increased on pressure; he had vomiting and much flatus, the stools were yellow and feculent, presenting nothing unnatural. Tongue covered with a yellowish brown fur. Flatulence was a constant and troublesome symptom. He died Dec. 7th. No mention is made of mercury having been administered.

Autopsy.—In the abdomen was about 7 pints of yellowish serum. In the upper and posterior part of the liver was an abscess, containing a large quantity of well formed pus; the peritoneum in many parts covered with coagulated lymph; in the stomach was a quantity of dark coloured fluid; the arch of the colon ulcerated in several places, and there were also many cicatrices of former ulcers. The caput coli had a sphacelated appearance; lungs healthy, with the exception of old adhesions to the diaphragm and ribs. (*Dr. Henderson*, ibid, *p.* 344.)

No. 41.—S. Smallman, æt. 33, 13 years in India, leuco-phlegmatic; had lived hard for 11 years, temperate for the last 2 years; admitted March 8th, with acute hepatitis, which, under depletion, purgatives, and the free use of mercurials, subsided. His convalescence, however, did not progress satisfactorily, and on April 18th, he complained of pain in the liver, increased by full inspiration and by pressure; tongue, white in the centre, with reddish tips and edges—pulse 92 small, skin moist. The subsequent symptoms were rigors attended with profuse sweats, vomiting, cough with a tickling sensation in the throat, much pain in the right lumbar region; the stools frothy and offensive, sometimes mucous, at others clay-coloured; the urine scanty and high coloured, or turbid, and latterly deposited a thick, white sediment. The abscess was opened on two occasions, with temporary benefit. He died May 23d, having for a few days previously passed some blood and pus, per anum.

Autopsy.—Liver enormous, filling the left hypochondrium, weighing 6 pounds; its substance pale, straw-coloured, and much softened. In the right lobe was an immense abscess, the surface of which was covered for a quarter of an inch with a layer of thick, indurated, unhealthy looking pus; on removing this, a false membrane of honey-combed structure was exposed underneath. Posteriorly and superiorly, the abscess had worked its way through the diaphragm into the cavity of the pleura, but was prevented discharging its contents, by a thick deposit of coagulable lymph; the matter was in contact with the intercostal muscles. The diaphragm itself was pushed up on a level with the mamma; the inferior lobe of the right lung adherent to the diaphragm; kidneys, normal; all the other abdominal viscera healthy. Case xxxiii, in List of Operations. (*Dr. W. R. Smyth*, ibid, vol. iii, *p.* 382.)

No. 42.—J. Lightfoot, æt. 25, 6 years in India, dissipated, repeatedly in hospital with hepatitis, and actively treated on each occasion; admitted with fatal attack April 14th, died May 11th, 1841, the abscess having been opened five days previously, to relieve the distressing dyspnæa. There was also enormous tympanitic distention of the abdomen. The history of the case not detailed.

Autopsy.—The right lobe of the liver converted into one large abscess, containing 3 pints of thick purulent matter; the walls were scarcely three lines in thickness, and were lined, to the extent of two inches, with a layer of thick curdy matter, which firmly adhered to the surface; left lobe healthy; the gall-bladder distended with thin fluid bile; the whole of the intestines glued together; on the mucous coat of the large intestines were numerous small pale ulcers. Stomach healthy; kidneys enlarged and pale. Case xxxiv, in List of Operations. (*Dr. W. R. Smyth*, ibid, vol. iii, *p.* 390.)

No. 43.—J. Myler, 20 years in India, feeble, most intemperate; admitted May 12th, with dysentery, which under treatment was nearly subdued, when, on the 17th, he complained for the first time, of pain in the right hypochondrium, increased on pressure, and attended by a short cough; pulse soft, skin cool and clammy. On the 21st, it is reported, "feels little or no pain in the side, but the pulse is frequent, with cold clammy perspirations, several scanty, watery motions in the night, slightly tinged with bile; feels extremely weak." He died on the 25th, having latterly made very little complaint of pain in the side. Treatment not given.

Autopsy.—Liver not much above the normal size, but converted into a mere shell, containing four abscesses, holding no less than 5 pints of pus. One was situated on the anterior surface of the right lobe, another on the concave surface, a third occupied the posterior part of the right lobe, and the fourth was in the centre of the left lobe. The remaining portion of the liver greatly congested, of a dark red colour, easily torn. Gall-bladder empty; mucous coat of the stomach indurated and thickened; small intestines inflated. The colon presented no morbid appearance. (*Dr. W. Parry, Madras Medical Journal*, vol. iv, *p.* 138.)

No. 44.—P. Kennedy, 3 years in India, a strong, robust, intemperate Irishman, admitted for the first time since he has been in India, July 20th, 1840, with severe pain in the abdomen, increased on pressure, particularly in the left hypochondrium, and in the course of the descending colon; frequent, scanty, watery stools, tinged with bile, but unmixed with blood; urgent tenesmus, and great irritability of the stomach. These symptoms continued unabated during the next two days, in spite of the most energetic treatment; it is not stated that he took mercury. On the 25th, the pain and tenderness had greatly subsided, but the other symptoms remained. He now became much exhausted, with cold clammy perspirations, hectic debility, and a rapid pulse. He died on the 31st, eleven days after admission. There was no pain in the shoulder; indeed, with the exception of the cold perspirations, there was no evidence during life, of hepatic abscess.

Autopsy.—Serous effusion into the abdominal cavity; the liver enlarged, softened, and of a deep colour; it contained four abscesses, one in the left, and three in the right lobe; the total quantity of matter was about two pints. Gall-bladder full of green bile, mucous coat of the stomach vascular, and in some places softened; the small intestines natural; the colon thickly studded throughout its inner surface with ulcers of various sizes; and near the caput coli, they were large and close, and covered with coagulated blood; one had perforated the intestine. (*Dr. W. Parry*, ibid, *p.* 139.)

No. 45.—M. Sheard, æt. 25, 1½ year in India, admitted Nov. 22d, 1841, with dysentery, accompanied by rigors and cold sweats. Under the use of depletives, mercury, &c. he improved. On Dec. 4th, he had pain in the region of the liver, increased by pressure; urine turbid, rigors and cold sweats. On the 11th, he passed purulent matter in his stools and urine, and this deposit continued copious for several days. He had also pain in the side and epigastrium, with dyspnæa, general soreness of the abdomen, œdema of the feet, evident enlargement of the side, anxious countenance, loss of appetite, sleeplessness, and a small rapid pulse. The liver was explored—coma supervened, and he died Dec. 6th.

Autopsy.—The whole of the right lobe of the liver studded with abscesses of various sizes, the largest deeply seated in the centre, containing a pint of thick, greenish, yellow pus; the smaller abscesses contained curdy matter. The left lobe was much indurated, and contained one small abscess. In the gall-bladder was a little dark inspissated bile. Large intestines extensively ulcerated; some of the ulcers gangrenous, and had perforated the coat of the intestine. Spleen enlarged and congested. (*Dr. Mouat,* ibid, vol. iv, *p.* 187.) This case is again quoted when considering the propriety of using the exploratory needle.

No. 46.—H. Neale, æt. 22, 1⅓ year in India, robust, intemperate, admitted January 16th, 1842, with purging of slime and blood, tenesmus and griping, severe pain at epigastrium and both hypochondriac regions, extending to the back, and much aggravated on pressure and inspiration. He was depleted, took calomel, ipecacuan, &c., with little or no benefit. Copious sweats, with a rapid pulse (120) supervened; fulness of the side now appeared, and the liver was explored; this gave some relief, but the cold sweats continued, and he died on the 28th. The stools throughout were brownish-red and watery, the urine, scanty, high coloured, and slightly turbid with deposit.

Autopsy.—Liver enlarged, pale, mottled; in the right lobe was one large abscess, partially filled with a slightly turbid serous fluid; no purulent matter was detected, till the substance of the viscus was broken down or compressed, when it exuded in a considerable quantity from the side of the cavity; the left lobe indurated; mesenteric glands enlarged; mucous coat of the stomach congested; small intestines much congested, and the large ones ulcerated throughout. Case xxxv, in List of Operations. (*Dr. Mouat,* ibid, *p.* 188.)

No. 47.—Capt. W. long ill, came under treatment April 27th, in a very weak state, a perfect skeleton, countenance anxious and ex-sanguineous, pulse small and rapid, tongue furred, skin natural. The treatment up to this date not given. The day previous, he vomited a coagulum of blood, six inches long and one thick, together with some dark, grumous blood. On examination, the liver was found enlarged, but he was not aware of any swelling of the side; he had, however, during his journey to Madras, felt occasional pain in the side, with pain in the shoulder, and numbness of the right arm, down to the wrist. He had previously one rigor, but never any unnatural or cold sweats; the bowels were irregular, and the stools latterly were black and offensive, and contained coagula of blood. He had excruciating burning in the stomach, especially after taking wine or beer, and he vomited, on several occasions, a quantity of black fluid like coffee grounds; a similar fluid was also passed by stool. The margin of the liver could be distinctly felt, about four inches below the ribs; at one point it presented an elasticity, but the remaining portion was hard and unyielding; the intercostal spaces were much increased. The right lobe was not painful on pressure, but there was tenderness in the left side over the stomach. He had constantly much flatulence, a great tendency to syncope, cold sweats, hurried breathing, and great debility. Delirium preceded death on the 30th Instant.

Autopsy.—Liver very large, occupying the entire epigastric region from rib to rib; the left lobe, and the Lobulus Spigelii were much enlarged, and harder than usual, but containing no abscess. The right lobe was occupied by one large abscess, containing about three quarts of purulent matter, serous fluid, and coagula of blood. The abscess-walls were hard, and nearly cartilaginous; in some parts they had a lacerated and ulcerated appearance; from this the blood had issued into the cavity of the abscess. The gall-bladder was healthy in structure, but distended, and contained a quantity of firmly coagulated blood, floating in a dark fluid, similar to that which was voided from the stomach and bowels, during life. A few small clots of blood was found adhering to the duodenum, but its coats were healthy; the small intestines healthy throughout; the stomach much contracted, having some small red spots, but no abrasion, on its mucous coat; cæcum thickened, and deeply ulcerated; in the ascending colon, also, were some points of ulceration. The spleen and pancreas, enlarged and hardened. On minute examination, no point in the stomach or intestines could be found, from which the blood, voided during life, could have oozed. It appears certain that the hæmorrhage must first have taken place into the sac of the abscess, and that the blood passed by the biliary vessels into the gall-bladder, thence into the duodenum. (*Samuel Rogers, Esq.*, ibid, vol. iv, *p. 393.*)

No. 48.—J. Hardacre, æt. 33, 8 years in India, admitted June 18th, 1839, with pain and swelling of the right side, increased by pressure and free respiration, frequent cough, scanty expectoration of mucus, dyspnæa, and difficulty of lying on the left side. Pulse 100 and small, skin dry and harsh, tongue furred, bowels irregular, frequently relaxed—has not been well for nearly two years. During the first night in hospital, he states that he felt something burst in his right side, and he expectorated a large quantity of purulent matter, mixed with coagula of blood: the fulness which he formerly complained of in the side, subsided at the same time. The expectoration of pus and blood continued, sometimes to the extent of a pint daily. He could not sleep, on account of the constant cough; pulse 100 to 120, feeble; skin moist; felt very weak, no appetite, much thirst. He died on the 28th, ten days after admission.

Autopsy.—Sero-purulent effusion into the abdominal cavity; a large abscess occupied the right lobe of the liver, pointing externally a little below, and to the right of the ensiform cartilage; a second had burst on the convex upper surface, and its contents passed through the lungs; a third pointed a little below, and to the right of the first; and a fourth had burst into the cavity of the peritoneum. About three quarts of pus were found in these abscesses. The left lobe and Lobulus Spigelii, only, intact; the other organs sound. (*A. B. Morgan, Esq.*, ibid, vol. iv, *p.* 397.)

No. 49.— ———, Admitted June 19th, 1837, with intermittent fever. He had a dry cough, fulness of the right side, which gradually increased; rigors and night sweats—fluctuation becoming evident, the abscess was opened, but the hectic continued, and he died 24 days after the operation.

Autopsy.—Liver of an enormous size, mottled, soft and granular, firmly adherent to the diaphragm, which was pushed upwards, encroaching on the chest. There were two large abscesses occupying the right and the middle lobes; the matter contained in them was of a bright orange colour, as if mixed with bile. State of the intestines not given. (*Dr. Stephenson, Mad. Med. Journ.* vol. v, *p.* 48.)

No. 50.—A scrofulous man of dissipated habits, admitted Sept. 7th, for the third time with hepatitis; he had severe pain in the right side extending to the right shoulder, oppressed respiration, slight fever, and depraved alvine secretions. He was depleted, blistered, and took occasional mercurial purgatives, but with little benefit; his countenance became pale and anxious, pulse 106 and small; he had pain between the two scapulæ, and could not lie down from fulness at the epigastrium; the right side was distended, and tender on pressure; urine red and turbid; the stools latterly became dysenteric, and attended with pain in the lower part of the abdomen. On October 9th, he coughed up about a pint of muco-purulent fluid, subsequently tinged with blood. Hectic fever, with œdema of the feet, and some delirium, supervened, and he died on the 26th, in a fit of syncope.

Autopsy.—The lower lobe of the right lung, adherent to the diaphragm, contained an abscess, the size of a hen's egg, which communicated, through an aperture in the diaphragm, with an abscess the size of an orange, in the right lobe of the liver; the latter was superficial, and its walls were broken down, and covered with dirty fetid pus. The liver was enlarged; the left lobe nearly equal in size to the right, and had an unctuous feel. The mucous coat of the large intestines congested, and towards the rectum, abrasions were observed. The right lung was much hepatized; the bronchial glands were enlarged, and filled with a melanotic deposit, which stained the fingers black. (*Dr. Nicholson*, ibid, vol. v, *p.* 86.)

No. 51.—J. Baillie, æt. 34. In this case, hepatic disease gradually supervened upon dysentery, and dissection disclosed a large abscess in the posterior surface of the right lobe of the liver. History not given. (*F. Dix, Esq.*, ibid, vol. v, *p.* 213.)

No. 52.—M. Connor, æt. 20, recently recovered from a chronic abscess between the abdominal muscles. Here, hepatic disease gradually supervened, whilst the man was in hospital for catarrh. Abscess in the liver was "suspected." History not given.

Autopsy.—An abscess was found in the upper surface of the liver, extending through the diaphragm into the right side of the chest. The abscess contained 16 ounces of pus. (*F. Dix, Esq.*, ibid, *p.* 214.)

No. 53.—W. Nelson, æt. 32. In this case, suppuration must have taken place before coming to hospital; he died four days after admission, though it was subsequently ascertained that he had been ill 12 or 14 days previously. Treatment not given.

Autopsy.—In the right lobe of the liver was a large abscess, which had burst through an opening in the diaphragm into the right pleural cavity; about 14 ounces of pus had escaped. (*F. Dix, Esq.*, ibid, *p.* 216.)

No. 54.—R. Flynn, æt. 34, 17 years in India, a ruddy coloured, healthy looking Irishman, of intemperate habits. Admitted July 16th, 1842, with hepatitis. He had a dull pain in the right side, which increased so much, that bleeding was necessary; he took calomel till his mouth became sore, when the pain subsided. Diarrhœa, and subsequently, dysentery supervened; improvement and relapse alternated, at times the stools being natural, and the pain in the side entirely gone. He became gradually emaciated, and the stools became bloody, serous, and highly offensive. He died Sept. 16th.

Autopsy.—The liver contained seven abscesses, the largest

being about the size of a large egg. The condition of the intestines not given. (*Dr. J. B. Preston*, ibid, vol. v, *p*. 250.)

No. 55.—R. Foreman, æt. 36, 16 years in India, a healthy looking Englishman, admitted July 16th, with hepatitis. He had very severe pain in the right hypochondrium, increased on pressure, and pain in the right shoulder. The tongue was foul and bilious, the pulse and skin natural. Next day, he had much dyspnæa, and his stomach became very irritable; from this time vomiting was a constant and distressing symptom; urine high coloured, stools dark and watery; tongue brownish yellow. The pain in the liver subsided under local depletion and calomel, and on the 22d there was no pain in the abdomen, even on heavy pressure; his countenance became shrunk, and he could retain nothing on his stomach. He died on the 26th.

Autopsy.—The right lobe of the liver contained two large abscesses. State of the intestines not given. (*D. J. B. Preston*, ibid, vol. v, *p*. 250—254.)

No. 56.—J. Spurway, æt. 33, a weak, sallow, unhealthy, intemperate man, admitted May 14th, 1841, with acute pain in the epigastric and hypochondriac regions, increased by pressure, and by lying on the right side; the liver was evidently much enlarged—and he had fever, with a small frequent pulse. He had been treated for dysentery, a few weeks previously, when he took mercury to the extent of affecting his mouth. Notwithstanding energetic treatment, the symptoms denoting abscess became apparent, as early as the sixth day, manifested by cold chills, clammy perspirations, emaciation, and anxeity of countenance. The liver was explored, but he got worse, and died on the 40th day after admission.

Autopsy.—The right lobe of the liver enormously enlarged, and contained four distinct abscesses, in one of which was 1½ pint of healthy pus. The condition of the other parts not stated. (*W. Parry, Esq*., ibid, vol. v, *p*. 321.)

No. 57.—P. Griffin, æt. 29, 1 year in India, admitted with intermittent fever Aug. 28th, and died Oct. 19th, 1840. History not given.

Autopsy.—Liver much enlarged, the right lobe closely adherent to the right side of the chest, contained a deep seated abscess, holding 10 ounces of purulent matter. The small intestines much injected at several places. The transverse arch of the colon much contracted, and its mucous coat in some places abraded, mesenteric glands enlarged, and of a purple colour. (*Dr. J, Middlemas*, ibid, vol. v, *p*. 364.)

No. 58.—J. Pyott, æt. 32, admitted Dec. 9th, 1837, with pain in the right hypochondrium, chest, and shoulder, attended by cough and dyspnæa; these symptoms left him in a few days, but he had still some uneasiness at the epigastrium. During January, his digestive organs were out of order, bowels sometimes relaxed, stools fluid and feculent, tongue furred, abdomen tumid, pulse irregular, sometimes intermittent. On the 30th, he passed two stools consisting of blood and pus, and next day he had another stool containing a great quantity of coagulated blood and pus; he was likewise seized with a cough, and expectorated muco-purulent matter; his abdomen now became full and distended, and he suffered from cold sweats and hiccough. He died February 1st. Treatment not given.

Autopsy.—Liver enlarged, weighing $6\frac{3}{16}$ pounds, soft, and of a yellow colour; the left lobe occupying the left hypochondrium; in the right lobe was an enormous abscess, which had burst through the diaphragm into the right lung. There were strong adhesions between the liver and diaphragm. The quantity of matter collected was $2\frac{1}{2}$ pounds. Serous effusion into the pericardium; the external surface of the heart granular, and of a vermillion colour. (*Dr. Watson, Mad. Med. Journ.* vol. vi, *p.* 22.)

No. 59.—M. Connor, æt. 29, admitted Jan. 29th, 1837, with pain in the region of the spleen, increased on coughing and respiring, a hot dry skin, and rapid pulse. These symptoms soon subsided, but his bowels remained relaxed, the stools vitiated, and, before death, mixed with blood. The abdomen was tumid, tongue dark, pulse quick, skin warm and dry. Latterly he was pretty free from pain, but the bowels were still relaxed. He died February 19th. Treatment not given.

Autopsy.—No visible fulness externally over the hepatic region, yet the liver was of an enormous size, weighing 6 pounds. There were strong adhesions between the liver and the abdominal parietes; the whole of the left lobe was converted into an abscess, containing 3 pounds of pus. In the right lobe were three distinct abscesses, holding altogether 5 pounds of pus. The large intestines, stomach, and spleen healthy. In the ilium was an intersusception—otherwise healthy. (*Dr. Watson,* ibid, vol. vi, *p.* 23.)

No. 60.—P. McGonnell, admitted Dec. 12th, 1836, with pain in the right hypochondrium shooting to the shoulder, cough, nausea, loss of appetite, and thirst; tongue furred, stools loose, semi-fluid, and slimy. As the disease progressed, the intensity of the pain became variable, and the number and nature of the stools irregular. Cough and night sweats supervened, and on the 7th Feb. he began to expectorate reddish purulent matter, and subsequently much pus, mixed with blood. The side was now swollen, and he had much pain and dyspnæa, attended by cold sweats, nausea, and sinking of the pulse. Towards the end of February the cough lessened, and the expectoration almost ceased, but the night sweats and rapid pulse continued. Diarrhœa supervened, and he died March 14th. Treatment not given.

Autopsy.—In the posterior part of the right lobe of the liver was the sac of a large abscess, communicating with the thorax, into which cavity 3 quarts of purulent matter had escaped. The right lung was compressed, and studded with small tubercles; the left lung healthy; the ascending colon thickened, and adherent to the peritoneum; the remaining portion of it, as well as the small intestines, stomach, and spleen healthy. (*Dr. Watson,* ibid, *p.* 25.)

No. 61.—T. Cruze, admitted March 11th, with pain in the right side stretching to the shoulder, pulse natural, tongue clean, bowels loose. In a few days the pain in the side entirely subsided, but the laxity of the bowels increased. His stools now became scanty, slimy, and bloody, attended with tenesmus and tormina, and a sense of weakness. The pulse became rapid, the tongue dry, furred, and dark, the skin cold and clammy. He died on the 22d. Treatment not given.

Autopsy.—The liver of its usual size, contained a small abscess in the superior part of the right lobe. In the abdominal cavity was effusion of dark brown fluid; in the colon were extensive ulcerations and abrasions, some of the ulcers had perforated the intestine; lungs and heart natural. (*Dr. Watson,* ibid, *p.* 25.)

No. 62.—S. Higgings, æt. 23, admitted Oct. 26th, with dysentery. On the 29th, his stools were thin and bilious, and he had pain in the right shoulder. On the 31st, he had pain in the right side, increased on inspiration. Next day the pain in the side was easier, but in the night, he had an increase of pain in the shoulder, with pyrexia; his tongue was now red and dry, the stools deficient of bile, the pain in the shoulder lessened, the stools sometimes semi-fluid and feculent, at others light yellow. On the 18th, the gums became tender, and he had increased pain in the side, augmented by pressure, and attended by much dyspnæa. On the 14th, he had a sudden attack of acute pain, the skin became cold and clammy, and he felt very weak; pulse 104 and feeble; stools semi-fluid, of a dark green colour; a fulness under the 7th and 8th ribs was now perceptible, but not to any great extent; the cold sweats continued, he became much emaciated, and died very suddenly, Nov. 21st. For some days prior to death, he had been expectorating greenish yellow sputa, the expectoration being difficult and scanty.

Autopsy.—The liver was adherent to the diaphragm, and at the superior portion of the right lobe a perforation had taken place, through which about 8 pints of pus, tinged with blood, had escaped; the abscess was situated in the superior portion of the liver, and was capable of holding an orange; the liver was enlarged, and pressed upon the stomach, the mucous coat of which was highly congested; the intestines, spleen, and kidneys, healthy; the right side of the thorax was completely filled with pus and serum, the right lung collapsed, the left healthy; heart healthy; pericardium contained a few ounces of clear serum. (*Dr. Watson*, ibid, vol. vi, *p.* 27.)

No. 63.—J. Evans, under treatment for hepatitis from the 10th to 15th April, 1843. History of the case not given.

Autopsy.—In the liver were ten distinct abscesses, having no connexion with each other; the whole colon was a mass of ulceration; the transverse arch immensely distended with gas. (*Dr. Gamble*, ibid, vol. vi, *p.* 96.)

No. 64.—D. A., æt. 34, 20 years in India, sallow complexion, temperate, very corpulent, admitted Aug. 17th, 1840, with feverishness unattended by pain, but the tongue was loaded, skin warm and dry, appetite defective, bowels irregular, urine free—pulse 96.

This officer had an abscess in the liver in 1838, and it was evacuated by operation, at the Cape of Good Hope in that year; he afterwards slowly recovered, and returned to India in 1839, since which time he enjoyed tolerably good health. "At present," says the report, "he is quite free from pain or uneasiness in the right side, and nothing unnatural can be detected on careful examination, though, from the corpulence of his person, it is difficult exactly to ascertain; there is no tension of the right rectus muscle perceptible.

Aug. 19th. Slept very well, bowels acting freely; feverish feeling removed, but the tongue is still white, the pulse still accelerated, skin cool and moist; complains of slight uneasiness near the sternal end of the clavicle on expiration, but not on inspiration. Appetite defective, thirst natural.

20th. Sense of languor and debility, stools dark coloured, offensive, urine free and natural; free from pain of any kind, tongue coated, skin cool, pulse 96.

21st. Occasional short cough, stools still dark; he is very sallow.

29th. Slept well, but this morning he complains of an uneasy feeling at the margin of the false ribs, and also at the top of the right shoulder on inspiring deeply; no fulness perceptible in the side, nor does pressure cause pain; urine free, stools dark but not offensive, skin cool, tongue clean, pulse 86.

Sept. 1st. Free from pain or any uneasiness in the right side; has occasional twitches about the clavicle, pulse and skin natural, appetite good.

12th. Caught a slight cold; has a sense of "stuffing" in the upper part of the chest, with a short cough, and pain in the pectoral muscles of the right side, otherwise tolerably well.

Oct. 1st. Evacuations, copious and watery, cough more frequent and troublesome, face swelled this morning, as well as the back of the hands, which are œdematous, pitting on pressure; a sense of stiffness in the thighs, urine free, pulse 94, tongue loaded, skin cool, but harsh and dry, lips ex-sanguineous, countenance sallow and unhealthy, side free from uneasiness. At 12 A. M. on this day, he suddenly felt an internal chill, followed by a sensation of something proceeding from the right hypochondrium to the umbilicus; he was bathed in a cold, clammy sweat, his countenance pale, sunk, and haggard; pulse 120, small and weak; voice hollow, severe griping pain at the umbilicus, and toward the pubes."

Although these severe symptoms subsided, he remained much debilitated, and the œdema extended, but he was almost constantly free from pain in the right side. He died Oct. 19th.

Autopsy.—Firm adhesions existed between the right lobe of the liver and the ribs. Particular attention was directed to the site of the former puncture, made for the evacuation of the abscess in 1838. Immediately opposite the external wound, the adhesions were very firm indeed, nearly of the consistence of cartilage; no cicatrix on the surface of the liver, nor mark of cavity of former abscess could be found, but this may perhaps be accounted for by the softened state of the liver. In the superior portion of the right lobe, was an abscess containing dark chocolate-coloured pus; the abscess had penetrated the diaphragm, and had become adherent to the middle lobe of the lung, in the lowest part of which was an abscess containing matter, similar to that above described. The portion of the lung surrounding, and immediately superior to the abscess, was quite hepatized, and apparently impervious to air, which may account for the absence of purulent expectoration at any stage of the disease; the coats of the sac were very thick and tough; the intestines and other abdominal viscera, healthy. (*Dr. M. B. Pollock,* ibid, vol. vi, *p.* 192.)

No. 65.—W. Oxenbold, æt. 18, admitted Oct. 4th, with hepatitis, and died Nov. 14th, 1841. History not given.

Autopsy.—In the upper surface of the liver was a large abscess, containing thick creamy pus; a fistulous opening led from this, through the diaphragm, into the right pleural cavity, which was partially filled with lymph and serum; the lung was collapsed, but not altered in structure; ulcerations existed in the upper part of the large intestines, and in the cæcum. (*Dr. McGregor,* ibid, vol. vi, *p.* 233.)

No. 66.—A native, a recruit in the 45th Regt. Madras Native Infantry, admitted at ½ past 9 A. M. complaining of pain in the right side, and of having had frequent calls to stool during the preceding night. Pulse small; skin cold and clammy; tongue furred; much emaciation. Mild stimulants were given, but he sank rapidly, and died at ¼ to 3 P. M., five hours and a quarter after admission.

Autopsy.—Firm adhesions existed between the whole of the upper surface of the right lobe of the liver and the diaphragm; on separating these carefully, a large abscess burst, containing 34 ounces of purulent matter; the lungs and all the other viscera appeared healthy. (*Dr. J. Kennedy,* ibid, vol. vi, *p.* 257.)

No. 67.—An European, æt. 21, steady, well-conducted, long in delicate health, admitted Sept. 14th, 1840, with fever and acute pain across the stomach, and in the right side, augmented by pressure. On the 15th, he had a severe rigor, and on the 20th, he voided by stool a large quantity of matter, slough, and coagulated blood. The pulse, which had been full and strong, became frequent and weak, and fluctuation being evident, the abscess was opened. He sank two days after, Sept. 22d.

Autopsy.—The liver was much enlarged; the right lobe gorged with blood, the left lobe was one large abscess, from which an opening had taken place into the colon; the liver was adherent to that viscus. Case lix, in List of Operations. (*Trans. of Med. and Phys. Society of Calcutta,* vol. v, *p.* 426.)

No. 68.—An European, æt. 26, admitted with fever, May 14th, 1830. On May 21st, for the first time, he had pain in the right side, and on the 24th, pain in the right shoulder. The treatment was most active; during the 4½ months he remained in hospital, he was bled four different times, to the amount, in all, of 68 ounces, and he had on 60 leeches; he took purgatives daily, as well as tartar emetic and calomel. Salivation was established 8 days after admission, and his mouth continued sore, nearly up to the time of his death. On July 27th, a sense of suffocation came on, and a copious expectoration of "phlegm;" the pulse becoming rapid, and the respiration hurried. Diarrhœa supervened, and he died Sept. 30th. There do not appear to have been any rigors, at any period of the disease.

Autopsy.—In the right lobe of the liver was a large abscess, with an opening from it into the lung. (*Ibid*, vol. v, *p*. 427.)

No. 69.—An European admitted August 14th, with fever, pain in the right side, and at the top of the shoulder. On the 22nd, ptyalism appeared, and his mouth remained sore for a long time. The treatment was as active as in the last case—bleeding, (to 64 ounces,) leeches, (60,) and blisters, (3,) besides issues. The chief symptoms were morbid heat of skin, pain in the right side, and in the front of the shoulder, with numbness extending to the arm and thigh. There was subsequently a sense of weight in the side, and the right ribs were observed to be heaved up—his pulse was frequent, and there was much feeling of faintness. The abscess burst into the thorax, apparently 7 days before death; at which period, in addition to great dyspnæa, he had obscure rigors. Diarrhœa supervened, under which he sunk, without having expectorated any matter.

Autopsy.—An enormous abscess in the liver was found to have made its way through the diaphragm into the right side of the chest. (*Ibid*, vol. v, *p*. 428.)

No. 70.—E. Beck, æt. 25, admitted May 1st, complaining of violent pain in the region of the liver and the præcordia; he had difficulty of lying on the left side, the tongue was foul, pulse full, eyes suffused with bile. The treatment was most energetic; he was bled four times to the amount of 130 ounces, had on 24 leeches, and used mercury externally till salivation was established—no benefit resulted; he continued to have pain, latterly of an obtuse character, augmented by pressure; he had likewise pain in the shoulder, rigors, much thirst, and loss of appetite; his countenance was sunk and cadaverous,—respiration difficult; there does not appear to have been vomiting at any period; bowels costive, only acted on by medicine, stools dark, loose, and offensive. Great debility, hectic, and night sweats preceded death on the 24th.

Autopsy.—Liver much enlarged, having in its centre an abscess containing several pints of matter; it had formed powerful adhesions to the diaphragm, through which it had discharged part of its contents into the pleural cavity, causing much inflammation. The whole of the alimentary canal was much indurated, and the blood vessels in a state of tergescence. The liver had formed no adhesion to the side. (*Surgeon Job, Madras Medical Reports, for* 1828, *p.* 398.)

No. 71.—J. Hamilton, æt. 37, 12 years in India—of healthy habit,—ill some weeks with dysentery,—admitted Nov. 5th, 1837, —passing blood and slime; skin cool, tongue white and loaded, appetite bad, abdomen flat and dull on percussion, some tenderness at the left extremity of the transverse arch, urine free. Latterly he had profuse sweats. Treatment consisted of calomel and opium, aperients, leeches to the anus, &c.

Autopsy.—Mucous membrane of the colon, thickened and ulcerated, interspersed with livid patches, particularly at the cæcum. Several small abscesses, some the size of an orange, throughout the liver, and the intervening substance soft, and of a pale yellow colour. Heart and lungs healthy. (*Dr. R. H. Hunter. Trans. of the Med. and Phys. Society of Bombay*, vol. ii, *p.* 33.)

No. 72.—J. Hannagan, æt. 36, 13 years in India, admitted with hepatitis, Jan. 3d, 1838. He had pain and tenderness in the epigastrium; pain in the back, shoulders, and loins; a dry cough, particularly at nights; aspect sickly, skin moderately warm, tongue loaded, thirst, anorexia, bowels open, pulse varying from 88 to 100; respiration high anteriorly, particularly on the left side, without deficiency of resonance, hepatic resonance from the 6th rib to an inch in front of the cartilaginous border; below that, abdominal and clear. Latterly much fulness of the side, night sweats, relaxed bowels, and great exhaustion. Seven days before death, on Jan. 18th, a deep incision over the most prominent part of the side, was made. Treatment, calomel and opium, latterly quinine, &c.

Autopsy.—Liver of an enormous size, of a dark blue colour, one small weak adhesion near the site of the incision; the right lobe full of thin green purulent matter, forming an immense abscess; the left lobe also enlarged, yellow, extremely lacerable, with here and there a small abscess the size of a bean. Lungs and intestines healthy. (*Dr. Hunter*, ibid, *p.* 26.)

No. 73.—D. McMay, sailor, admitted Aug. 26th, 1838; ill for some months. The symptoms on admission were bulging of the right side, emaciation, loose bowels with grey coloured stools; the skin was yellow and dry, tongue red and streaked with yellow, pulse soft, abdomen collapsed. On Oct. 7th, he had a cough with expectoration of viscid yellow mucus, tickling uneasiness at the top of the larynx, and oppressed breathing; pulse 108, small and feeble. There was also protrusion of the ribs on the right side, from the fourth downwards; dull sound on percussion, respiratory murmur not audible, except at the upper part, where it was accompanied by a mucous râle; bronchophony under the right clavicle, respiration of the left side, peurile. He died Oct. 24th. The treatment consisted of counter-irritation, occasional mercurials, with quinine and opium.

Autopsy.—The liver dark coloured and softened; in the right lobe, which was adherent to the diaphragm, was an abscess the size of an orange, which had made its way through the diaphragm, and had discharged about 4½ pints of greenish purulent matter into the right thoracic cavity; in the stomach were some abraded spots, in other parts it was thickened and mammilated; the lower end of the ilium was thickened, and of a pearly hue; similar changes were observed in the colon and cæcum; there were cicatrices of ulcers throughout the large intestines, and likewise some patches of granular lymph. Mesenteric glands enlarged, kidneys dark congested, spleen firmly adherent to the side, much serous effusion into the abdominal cavity. (*Dr. J. Bird, Trans. of the Med. and Phys. Society of Bombay*, vol. ii, *p.* 86.)

No. 74.—T. Saunders, æt. 36, stout habit, recently from England, admitted Aug. 9th, 1838, with pain in the head, side, and limbs; he had also cough, and the pain in the side was increased by inspiration; ill 5 days. On admission he was dull of hearing, his manner slow and undecided, and his hands were frequently tremulous; spirits depressed, pulse excited. Sept. 1st, "still nervous, but makes no complaint of the side; there is, however, a greater fulness of the right hypochondrium than of the left, and the nipple is on a lower level than that of the left side. About two inches below the right nipple, and laterally and posteriorly below the inferior angle of the scapula, there is dulness on percussion; the respiratory murmur is obscure, with occasional sibilus and crepitation. On the left side of the chest there is occasional sibilus and mucous ronchus; there is no cough." Subsequently the cough became troublesome, and the pulse frequent. On the 16th, he became drowsy, then insensible, and died at 7 P. M. *Treatment.* Leeches, warm baths, blisters, mercurials, quinine, and aperients, which were required to keep the bowels open.

Autopsy.—An abscess of considerable size in the right hemisphere of the brain, the surrounding substance softened; the liver was red and softened, and adhered to the ribs and diaphragm;

on separating the latter adhesion, a small abscess was discovered, and opposed to it, the right lung; of this the lowest lobe was much hepatized, and the left lung congested with blood. (*Dr. C. Morehead*, ibid, vol. ii, *p.* 110.)

No. 75.—W. Morris, æt. 63, sailor, admitted Aug. 5th, 1838, having been ill 8 days with pain in the right hypochondrium and shoulder; he also had cough; the bowels were constipated, the urine scanty, tongue rough and furred. On the 7th, these symptoms were improved, the pulse and skin were natural, and he inspired freely; but he was much depressed in spirits, and had an uncomfortable feeling in the chest and epigastrium; next day he winced under pressure at the margin of the right false ribs, and there was some fulness of the abdomen. On the 12th, the tongue was dryish, the stools scanty and tinged with blood, the eyes were suffused and heavy, and he continued much depressed in spirits. Little change took place till the 17th, when the respiration was hurried; there was acute pain in the abdomen, a purplish tinge of the face and surface, cold skin, and feeble pulse. The pain continued excruciating, and he was constantly moaning till his death, which took place the same night. Treatment. Leeches, calomel, occasionally; purgatives, blisters, &c.

Autopsy.—Liver not enlarged, its substance dark and indurated; it adhered firmly to the diaphragm, and on attempting a separation, an abscess was found, apparently immediately below the peritoneal covering, containing puriform serum; the stomach showed marks of inflammatory action; the mucous coat of the small intestine healthy; that of the colon, dark-grey with speckles of red, thin, and in some places almost removed. There was sero-puriform effusion into the abdominal cavity, with general peritonitis. There was also serous effusion at the base of the brain, and in the ventricles. (*Dr. C. Morehead*, ibid, vol. ii, *p.* 126.)

No. 76.—J. Harrison, æt. 33, 13 years in India, slight made, admitted Feb. 25th, 1839, with pain and tenderness in the right iliac region, where there was a defined knotty hardness, emitting a dull sound on percussion; this pain extended to the margin of the false ribs of the same side. The pulse was generally from 80 to 88, feeble, often thready, skin cold and damp, tongue moist and without fur; 2 or 3 yellow watery evacuations were passed daily. He died March 5th. Treatment. Quinine with Hyd. e Cretâ, and palliatives.

Autopsy.—The liver of the natural size, mottled, and of a pale fawn colour, except around two or three small abscesses in the right lobe, where the mottling was dark-red; no ulceration of the large intestine; stomach and thoracic viscera healthy; sero-purulent effusion in the abdominal cavity. (*Dr. Morehead*, ibid, vol. ii, *p.* 132.)

No. 77.—A. Lopes, æt. 42, a Portuguese sailor, admitted Jan. 22, 1839, having been ill for 20 days with dysentery; his countenance was sallow and anxious, the abdomen tender and tense, with tenderness on pressure over the cæcum, pulse feeble, tongue expanded and a little furred. On the 23d, there was distinct defined hardness felt over the cæcum; the bowels continued loose, the stools watery, greenish or light-yellow, the tongue generally pretty clean, the pulse rarely above 76; the tumour over the cæcum continued distinct till Feb. 2d, when the tenderness and the fulness of the abdomen became more general. He died on the 7th instant. Treatment. Leeches, blisters, blue pill or calomel, with ipecacuanha and opium, latterly quinine and opium.

Autopsy.—The omentum crossed from the 9th or 10th false ribs, adhered to the anterior parietes, passed obliquely to the hollow of the right os ilium, and thus divided the cavity into two parts; the upper contained a pint of pus, in a circumscribed sac, lined with false membrane; the lower division contained two pints of serum, with flakes of lymph. The small intestines were much inflamed and matted together; the cæcum adhered firmly to the omentum, and to the hollow of the os ilium; there were round isolated ulcerations, here and there, in the colon; the liver was much enlarged, and in the right lobe was a large abscess with a firm lining membrane; the parenchyma was of a dark-red colour, and mottled white; the left kidney was in a state of yellow degeneration. (*Dr. Morehead*, ibid, vol. ii, *p.* 134.)

No. 78.—G. Dunn, æt. 38, of spare habit, admitted Aug. 6th, 1838; he was deaf, articulated indistinctly, and was evidently labouring under disease of the brain. Amongst other measures, the action of mercury was induced mildly on the system. On the 17th of October, he had, for the first time, tenderness of the abdomen, with diarrhœa. On the 25th, there was fulness and tenderness at the epigastrium and the right side. He gradually got worse, and died Nov. 8th.

Autopsy.—Much serous effusion was found in the head, with much thickening of the arachnoid. In the left lobe of the liver was an abscess, the size of an orange; the right lobe healthy; there was general peritonitis, with some sero-purulent effusion into the abdominal cavity; in the colon were a few round ulcers, and some dark-grey cicatrices; stomach mottled, but neither thickened nor softened; both kidneys had undergone yellow degeneration to a considerable extent; the lungs healthy. (*Dr. Morehead*, ibid, vol. ii, *p.* 135.)

No. 79.—J. Williams, æt. 28, sailor, admitted May 20th, 1838, with acute pain at the scrobiculus cordis, increased by pressure, and attended with febrile excitement. On the 22d, the pain had extended to the right hypochondrium, augmented by deep inspiration, and by decubitus on the left side. Under the use of V. S., leeches, blisters, purgatives, and mercury till the gums were tender, he greatly improved, and complained only of weakness. On the 30th, he had rigors, followed by febrile excitement, and recurrence of pain in the side. On June 1st, 2d, 3d, and 4th, there was an evening febrile exacerbation; the subsequent symptoms were frequent night sweats, emaciation, occasional pain in the side, with a tickling cough and feeble pulse; sometimes decubitus on the left side caused uneasiness, and sometimes not; there was no enlargement below the edge of the right false ribs, but there was slight bulging of the ribs themselves, and a want of depression of the intercostal spaces. The physical signs made it clear that the right side of the chest was much encroached upon, laterally as high as the axilla, and anteriorly to the level of the nipple; the sound was quite dull on percussion, and the respiratory murmur was inaudible. Latterly there was much vomiting, but nothing ejected except ingesta, and the mucous secretions of the stomach. At no period was there diarrhœa, or dysentery; on the contrary laxatives were often required, and generally, but more especially latterly, the evacuations were *formed* and perfectly natural. He died Sept. 5th.

Autopsy.—The liver adherent to the side and diaphragm; the whole of the right lobe was completely occupied by a large abscess, containing serous fluid at the upper surface, and purulent matter below, in all about 4 pounds; the sac was lined by a firm cartilaginous membrane, to which yellow flocculi adhered. A thin layer of parenchyma interposed between the peritoneal covering, and the sac was of dense cellular tissue, about half an inch thick; the left lobe mottled, the diaphragm pushed up on a level with the 2d rib; the right lung collapsed and crepitating; the gall-bladder contained some bile; the stomach and intestines almost natural, and the colon partially occupied with formed and perfectly natural feculence; kidneys healthy; there was some serous effusion at the base of the brain. (*Dr. Morehead*, ibid, vol. ii, *p.* 136.)

No. 80.—J. Taylor, æt. 42, 13 years in India, slight habit, ill for 5 days with irritability of the stomach, and occasional flushes of heat; admitted Oct. 24th, 1838; he had much tenderness on pressure, below the margin of the right false ribs, and had easiest decubitus on the right side; the tongue was furred in the centre, pulse 84, skin perspiring. The pain in the side subsided for a time, but it returned on the 26th, and extended into the right iliac region, being augmented by motion and slight pressure; pulse 76, soft; the stools dark-brown and watery. Little change took place till the 29th, when there was added a want of suppleness on pressing the tender part of the abdomen. The pulse ranged from 90 to 112, and was soft and feeble; the stools watery, with red flocculi, and passed without straining; the pain continued more or less, and on Nov. 1st, there was distinct fulness under the right rectus muscle. Mercury failed to affect the system. Slight delirium preceded death, Nov. 4th.

Autopsy.—The omentum adherent to the edge of the liver, and to the small intestines; on separating these adhesions, the coats of the cæcum and colon readily tore away, and showed their mucous coat covered with large sloughing ulcerations; the sigmoid flexure of the colon and the rectum were the only healthy parts of the large intestines; the liver adhered to the ribs, the diaphragm, and the stomach, and its substance was studded with abscesses about the size of walnuts, each with a membranous bag; the thoracic viscera healthy. (*Dr. Morehead*, ibid, vol. ii, *p.* 139.)

No. 81.—A gentleman, of full habit, æt. 46, 27 years in India, subject to attacks of gout and rheumatism, swelling of the joints, and also to the repeated occurrence of obstinate constipation. About two months before admission, he was attacked with diarrhœa, alternating with constipation, and scybalous discharges. On admission, (April 17th, 1835,) he was much reduced in flesh, his countenance anxious and languid, tongue florid, bowels relaxed, stools dark-green, watery, offensive, and there was tenderness on pressure in the right iliac region. The treatment not given. Occasional drowsiness, increasing weakness, and vomiting of inky coloured fluid preceded death, May 2d.

Autopsy.—The stomach much distended with dark, inky fluid; but, with the exception of softening of some points, the mucous coat was healthy. There was an abscess in the right iliac region, bounded in part by the concave surface of the liver, the fundus of the gall-bladder, a portion of the omentum, the ascending colon and the right kidney; this purulent deposit communicated with an extensive but very superficial abscess, on the inferior surface of the liver, to the right of the Lobulus Spigelii; the descending colon was contracted, and the sigmoid flexure was about the diameter of a swan's quill; there were no ulcerations, but there were traces of cicatrices in the cæcum and ascending colon, the mucous coats of which were thickened, and presented black mottled patches; the small intestines filled with dark-green viscid fluid. (*Dr. Morehead,* ibid, vol. ii, *p.* 141.)

No. 82.—T. Dean, æt. 22, sailor, admitted Jan. 18th, 1839, ill 2 months with hepatitis, for which he had been actively treated and taken blue pill, ipecacuanha, &c. He was now pale but not emaciated, had night sweats and cough, with expectoration of brick-red puriform sputa. On percussion, there was dulness as high as the 4th rib, and subsequently as high as the axilla of the right side. The sputa continued copious, the pain in the right side was sometimes complained of, and the position in which he suffered least, was resting on the left side, and bending forwards; tongue clean, moist, pulse 100, bowels occasionally relaxed. On April 2d, there was an increase of pain in the right side, which subsequently extended over the abdomen; it was increased by pressure, and by lying down, so that he was obliged to remain in a sitting posture. The abdomen now became very distended, the pulse feeble, the countenance collapsed, but the cough and expectoration decreased. He died suddenly, on the 12th Instant.

Autopsy.—Serous effusion into the abdominal cavity, agglutination of the small intestines—*some of the convolutions of the ilium passed over the hepatic flexure of the colon, and were interposed between the liver and the ribs.* The liver was adherent, at one point, to the diaphragm, through which a superficial abscess had discharged itself into the right sac of the pleura. The lowest lobe of the right lung adhered to the diaphragm, and was in part converted into a sac filled with purulent matter. The liver reached to the 3d rib, and the contents of the abscess seemed to have escaped into the pleura, to have been circumscribed by adhesions, and thence discharged through the lung. (*Dr. Morehead, Trans. of Med. and Phys. Society of Bombay,* vol. vii, *p.* 38.)

No. 83.—J. Roberts, æt. 29, of feeble habit, was under treatment for acute hepatitis from April 30th, to May 16th, 1839; on this occasion he was bled freely, and took calomel, but not to ptyalism. He was re-admitted June 5th, with diarrhœa, which resisted all treatment. On July 3d, distinct hardness and tumefaction between the margin of the right ribs and the os ilium was first noted; blisters were frequently applied, but without benefit.

He continued to lose ground, became much emaciated and sallow, and on August 3d, it is noted for the first and only time, that he had been much troubled with cough during the previous night. He died on the 24th Instant.

Autopsy.—The right lobe of the liver extended three inches below the margin of the ribs, and the edge of the lobe, to the right of the gall-bladder, was occupied by an abscess, the size of an orange, with dense fibrous walls. The hepatic flexure of the colon, and part of the omentum, were matted to the walls of this abscess. Close to the diaphragm, also in the right lobe, was another abscess, the lobe itself being adherent to the diaphragm; the rest of the surface of the liver was mottled white. The mucous coat of the cæcum was studded with small follicular ulcerations, some of them cicatrizing; the mucous coat of the colon was nearly healthy. Both kidneys were enlarged. At the base of the brain, and also in the pericardium, the right thorax and the abdominal cavity, serous effusion had taken place. (*Dr. Morehead*, ibid, vol. vii, *p.* 35.)

No. 84.—R. Dunstan, æt. 39, 2 years in India, ill several days, much reduced in flesh, admitted January 16th, 1841, with uneasiness at the epigastrium, not amounting to pain, and not increased either by pressure, full inspiration, or by decubitus on either side; the skin was moist, pulse 112, feeble and easily compressed. He continued languid and depressed, with collapsed and anxious countenance, a quick feeble pulse and a brownish tongue, sometimes dry in the centre; the bowels were generally moved daily, but scantily; but on the 23d he passed by stool, more than a pint of coagulated blood. He died early on the following morning.

Autopsy.—The liver filled both hypochondria; the right lobe was adherent to the diaphragm, and contained two large abscesses; the left lobe healthy. There were patches of vascularity in the stomach. The colon contained some dark, claret-red slimy fluid, its mucous coat had throughout a reddish tinge, and presented several patches of ulceration. The lowest lobe of the right lung, adherent to the diaphragm; the left lobe, and also the heart, were healthy. In the right sac of the pleura was effusion of 30 ounces of sero-purulent fluid. (*Dr. Morehead*, ibid, vol. vii, *p.* 36.)

No. 85.—J. Shea, æt. 28, admitted into hospital Nov. 22d, 1840, in a moribund state, and died eight hours after admission. He had first been taken ill with hepatitis on the 6th of August; under treatment, he improved, but the disease recurred severely on the 23d of the same month. There was severe pain in the hepatic region, increased by decubitus on the left side, and by pressing the liver against the diaphragm. On the 6th of October, he was suddenly seized with expectoration of purulent matter, which continued till the period of his death.

Autopsy.—The right lung was slightly adherent to the ribs and diaphragm; in the upper lobe were a few tubercles; it was very œdematous and in parts hepatized; in the lowest lobe was an abscess the size of an orange, which communicated, through the diaphragm, with an abscess in the upper part of the right lobe of the liver, about the same size; it was superficial, and had a firm lining membrane, with an irregular flocculent surface. The rest of the liver was healthy. On the surface of the heart were many white pearly spots, but the organ was sound. In the colon were a few small, circular ulcers, and the cicatrices of many others. The kidneys and spleen were healthy. (*Dr. Morehead*, ibid, vol. vii.)

No. 86.—S. Cain, æt. 50,—ill eight days—admitted Jan. 24th, 1840, with pain in the right side, shooting from the margin of the ribs to the shoulder. On Feb. 4th, there was tenseness, fulness, and hardness at the margin of the right ribs; on the 7th, the breathing became oppressed, and there was general distention of the abdomen, with pain from time to time. He died on the 14th Instant.

Autopsy.—The liver projected two or three inches beyond the margin of the ribs, and there was an abscess about the size of an orange, circumscribed, chiefly between the diaphragm and the upper surface of the liver; the peritoneal surface of the intestines was dark-red; the convolutions were united by flakes of lymph, and sero-purulent fluid was effused among them; the mucous coat of the stomach was of a dark, leaden-grey colour; there were 5 pounds of pus in the right pleural cavity, but it is not stated that any communication existed between it and the abscess. (*Dr. Morehead*, ibid.)

No. 87.—A. McLean, æt. 32, a few months in India,—subject to hepatitis,—ill four days with dysenteric symptoms; admitted Dec. 27th, 1840, with tenderness at the epigastrium and margin of the right ribs, painful decubitus on the left side, nausea, and an excited pulse. He was freely depleted, and calomel was given ineffectually, with the view of inducing ptyalism. He died on the 10th of January.

Autopsy.—The liver was adherent to the small arch of the stomach; in both lobes were several abscesses, the largest the size of an orange; they did not form distinct sacs, but seemed to consist of a breaking down of the parenchyma by purulent infiltration into the cellular tissue, which connects the ramifications of the terminal cæca of the secretory substance; the large intestines were partially ulcerated. (*Dr. Morehead*, ibid, vol. vii, *p*. 38.)

No. 88.—R. Cox, sailor, æt. 46, admitted Feb. 4th, 1841: he had been ill 7 days with a dry cough, attended with pain in the lower part of the chest, extending to the epigastrium, and increased by pressure; pulse frequent, skin dry. He was freely depleted, and took calomel in ten grain doses, but without affecting his mouth. The pain never ceased, although partially relieved, purging set in, the skin became washy, the pulse feeble, the countenance collapsed, and he died on the 12th Instant.

Autopsy.—On the lateral part of the right lobe of the liver was a superficial abscess, containing a dark, reddish serous fluid; its walls yellow and flocculent. About the anterior part of the right lobe, was a yellow substance, the size of a walnut, softened in the centre, firmer beyond, (an incipient abscess?) The substance of the liver was mottled buff; the colon presented a dark-red surface, covered with a yellow granular firm secretion, and frequent traces of inflammation; there was yellow deposit in one of the kidneys. (*Dr. Morehead*, ibid, vol. vii, *p*. 39.)

No. 89.—J. Martin, æt. 39, admitted February 2d, 1841—ill 14 days with dysentery, and pain with tenderness across the abdomen. Subsequently the pain was chiefly about the margin of the right ribs, shooting downwards to the iliac region, and also into the epigastrium, and there was distinct fulness and tenderness at the margin of the ribs. On the 4th, there was a distinct febrile paroxysm with rigor. On the 12th, he passed much brick-red puriform matter, which continued till his death on the 14th Inst. At first the case was treated as dysentery, but when it was clear that the liver was chiefly affected, an attempt was made to induce the action of mercury on the system, but it caused irritation, and was not persisted in. Leeches, blisters, and, latterly, wine with quinine and opium, were employed.

Autopsy.—In the liver, to the right of the gall-bladder, was a large abscess, which at one point was adherent to the colon, but no communication was found to exist; a second abscess, the size of an orange, was found in the right lobe; the contents of both, were dark-brown, quite serous, the walls in each case consisting of broken down flocculent substance. The other portion of the liver had a bright buffed, mottled appearance. On the mucous coat of the colon were numerous superficial extensive ulcerations. Lungs emphysematous, otherwise healthy. (*Dr. Morehead*, ibid, vol. vii, *p*. 40.)

No. 90.—T. Conolly, æt. 40, sailor, of slight habit, ill 4 days, admitted March 24th, 1841, with acute pain in the right side, and frequent purging; the pain prevented full inspiration, and extended downwards to the iliac region; pulse 100, sharpish, but easily compressed, skin moist, tongue coated in the centre, and florid at the tip. He was bled locally and generally, but he bore the depletion badly, and the pain continued unabated. Subsequently, there was frequent vomiting, and fulness and tenseness, extending from the margin of the ribs to the right iliac fossa; the left side was supple. He died on the 30th. The treatment was chiefly palliative—calomel only on two occasions.

Autopsy.—The omentum adhered in places to the intestines, and also to the edge of the right lobe of the liver. There was a portion of the substance of the liver, the size of a large orange, at the thin part of the right lobe, of a white colour, in parts tolerably firm, in others pulpy, and in others breaking down into pus—bounded by a firm sac, from which the white part could be scraped; and over this portion of the liver was a circumscribed abscess, bounded by the abdominal parietes, the omentum, and the liver; the hepatic tissue was mottled red and white; the colon was contracted, with ulcers, here and there, on its mucous coat. Lungs emphysematous. (*Dr. Morehead*, ibid, *p.* 41.)

No. 91.—J. Richards, Indo-Briton, æt. 26, ill 21 days, admitted Jan. 29th, 1841, with pain in the right side, preventing full inspiration and decubitus on the right side. He was depleted, and though mercury was used externally and internally, nothing but a swollen state of the gums was induced; the pain was relieved, but not removed entirely, no fulness at the margin of the ribs was observed, nor rigors, at any period of the disease. On February 1st, dysenteric symptoms supervened, (apparently following the exhibition of a seven grain dose of calomel,) and the tenesmus for some days was urgent. Latterly the bowels were moved 7 or 8 times in the 24 hours, the stools being watery and brown. He lost flesh, and died on the 17th.

Autopsy.—The liver did not extend beyond the ribs; the lateral part of the right lobe adherent to the ribs, and underneath this adhesion, was an abscess, the size of an ostrich egg, containing 20 ounces of thick pus; it was lined by a firm cartilaginous membrane, beyond which, for 3 or 4 lines, the parenchyma was cartilaginous and condensed. From the surface of the lining of the sac, loose flocculi depended, and were easily scraped off with a knife. In both lobes were several round, yellow-buff, defined portions, from the size of a tare to that of a horse-bean, some consistent throughout, others with a drop of pus in the centre; the mucous coat of the colon was pale, with traces of ulcers in the process of cicatrization; the right lung emphysematous, and adherent to the diaphragm; kidneys and heart, healthy. (*Dr. Morehead*, ibid, *p*. 41.)

No. 92.—J. McInnis, Engineer, æt. 33, ill ten days, admitted April 12th, 1841, with hepatitis. On the 20th, there was unexpected collapse with vomiting. He continued till his death, on the 30th, to suffer from occasional vomiting, and hiccup; latterly the abdomen was full, with pain shifting from place to place; pulse frequent.

Autopsy.—Liver adherent to the ribs; in the right lobe were two abscesses; sero-purulent effusion had taken place in the abdominal cavity, and there was slight agglutination of portions of the intestines; the gall-bladder showed marks of inflammation; it was moderately distended, and adherent to the colon; the stomach had a rosy tint, but was unchanged in structure. (*Dr. Morehead*, ibid, vol. vii, *p*. 43.)

No. 93.—D. Hopkirk, sailor, æt. 26, admitted Dec. 16th, 1840, with intermittent fever, (with which he had been ill for 21 days,) and pain in the upper part of the abdomen, increased on pressure; subsequently this pain only recurred occasionally, together with febrile paroxysms and rigors; dysenteric purging and loss of flesh preceded death, on Feb. 9th, 1841. He was depleted, and though he took mercury freely, he was not brought under its influence. At one time he had clavus hystericus, the result, probably, of the active depletory measures.

Autopsy.—Liver red and firmer than usual; the right lobe was adherent to the side, and at this point, contained a superficial abscess, the size of an ostrich egg, lined with a firm smooth membrane; around this, in the substance of the liver, were several tubercles, the size of a pin's head, and in the centre of the right lobe, was one the size of a horse-bean; the colon and cæcum in a state of sloughing ulceration; their coats black and friable. Mesenteric glands enlarged; kidneys in a state of yellow degeneration; lungs emphysematous; heart healthy. (*Dr. Morehead*, ibid, vol. vii, *p*. 43.)

No. 94.—T. Hall, æt. 32, ill 21 days, admitted with hepatitis, Jan. 10th, 1840. Within nine days after admission, his gums were sore from mercury. He had pain in the right side, shooting towards the nipple of that side, short cough, febrile exacerbations, and increasing emaciation. On March 6th, general fulness at the margin of the right rib was apparent. He died on the 15th.

Autopsy.—Liver very large, extending upwards as high as the 3d rib, and downwards for two inches below the costal cartilages. In the right lobe was an abscess containing 3 pounds of thick pus, its upper wall consisting merely of the diaphragm and the peritoneal coat of the liver; the cardiac end of the stomach was mottled red; the mucous coat of the large intestines was dark-red and dark-grey, but not ulcerated; lungs collapsed; effusion of serum at the base of the brain. (*Dr. Morehead*, ibid, vol. vii, *p.* 44.)

No. 95.—J. Robinson, sailor, æt. 26, admitted Sept. 7th, 1840, with hepatitis, for which he was bled freely, and used mercury externally and internally, but without inducing ptyalism. On the 12th, he began to have evening febrile exacerbations, and on the 15th, there was fulness at the margin of the ribs, with hepatic sound, from an inch below them to within two inches of the right nipple; the fulness of the side increased, he became sallow and emaciated, the breathing was oppressed, the stools thin and light-yellow. He died on the 22d.

Autopsy.—Liver enlarged, extending as high as the 4th rib, not adherent to the diaphragm; in the right lobe, were several abscesses, the size of an orange, with flocculent walls, the flocculi floating in water; the left lobe filled the left hypochondrium, was of a pale colour, and presented white defined portions, the size of a pea, like tubercles in appearance, but not so hard in texture. Of the above abscesses, two were on the concave surface of the liver, and closely adherent to the colon; this intestine, on its mucous coat, was closely studded with circular ulcers, some of them in a sloughing state; in the ilium, granular lymph was effused; the lungs were emphysematous, and there was slight serous effusion at the base of the skull. (*Dr. Morehead*, ibid, *p.* 45.)

No. 96.—W. Sonarry, æt. 35, admitted April 9th, with hepatitis, of which he had had several previous attacks. From May 1st to the period of his death, (June 21st,) there was more or less cough, with much grey puriform expectoration.

Autopsy.—A large abscess occupied the right lobe of the liver, and there were several abscesses on the convex surface; in the colon were transverse ridges of ulceration; lungs natural. (*Dr. Morehead*, ibid, *p.* 46.)

No. 97.—G. Bignell, æt. 28, 9 months in India, ill 3 days, admitted Jan. 2d, 1840, with pain in the right side, shooting to the shoulder, and impeding full inspiration. V. S., leeches, and blisters were used, and he was brought mildly under the influence of mercury. He did not convalesce satisfactorily; and on the 29th, there was return of pain in the side, and the liver was distinctly felt, two inches below the ribs; the fulness of the side, subsequently, became more distinct, and there was hepatic sound almost to the nipple; the tongue coated and florid at the tip; emaciation, hectic, and diarrhœa preceded his death, Feb. 26th.

Autopsy.—Liver adherent to the ribs; a circumscribed abscess existed between the surface of this viscus and the side; the liver extended 3 inches below the margin of the ribs, and in the upper part of the right lobe was an abscess, the size of a hen's egg, with flocculent walls; the mucous coat of the stomach, red-brown, but normal in structure; that of the large intestines presented a surface of closely set circular ulcers, in places running into each other; right lung adherent to the diaphragm. (*Dr. Morehead,* ibid, *p.* 46.)

No. 98.—A. Annesley, æt. 31, ill a long time with hepatitis, from which he had never completely recovered; admitted Jan. 5th, 1840, and died Jan. 26th. He was sallow and thin, had pain in the right side, a short cough, and general fulness of the abdomen, with obscure fluctuation. Latterly there was increased cough and diarrhœa, and distinct prominence at the margin of the right ribs.

Autopsy.—Liver much enlarged, with a large abscess in the right lobe, containing 3½ pounds of pus; there were two smaller abscesses at the edge of the liver; mucous coat of the intestines thinned, with granular secretion on that of large intestines. (*Dr. Morehead,* ibid, *p.* 47.)

No. 99.—W. Harris, æt. 23, admitted with a relapse of hepatitis, Oct. 10th, 1841. On the 28th, expectoration of brick-red sputa commenced, which continued till the date of his death, on Feb. 1st. Tumefaction, with fluctuation, being evident, the abscess was opened Dec. 15th, and brick-red puriform discharge, with air, passed from the wound.

Autopsy.—The orifice between the 7th and 8th ribs enlarged from sphacelus; the subjacent tissue and intercostal muscles, for about the extent of two inches, removed by sphacelus; the 7th rib was in a state of caries, and in consequence was fractured near the junction with the cartilage; the abscess in the liver was very superficial, bounded by the convex part of the right lobe, the diaphragm, and the ribs; the base of the third lobe of the right lung adhered to the diaphragm, and at its anterior part there was an excavation, the size of a walnut, which communicated with the sac of the abscess; there were old adhesions of the surface of the liver, and also of the omentum to the abdominal parietes; lungs collapsed and crepitating. Case lxx, in List of Operations. (*Dr. Morehead*, ibid, vol. vii, *p.* 47.)

No. 100.—W. Campbell, æt. 37, ill a week, admitted Oct. 27th, 1841, with tenderness and fulness of the epigastrium, irritability of the stomach, and thirst; he was emaciated and sallow, skin hot and dry, tongue and hands tremulous, but he denied having been drinking freely. He had also a frequent, short cough, more or less without expectoration; the tumefaction of the epigastrium also became prominent and tense; no diarrhœa. The treatment was chiefly palliative.

Autopsy.—The right lobe of the liver was completely occupied with an abscess containing sero-purulent fluid; the sac of the right pleura also filled with similar fluid; no communication is stated to have existed. (*Dr. Morehead*, ibid, vol. vii, *p.* 48.)

No. 101.—A. Scott, æt. 72, a pensioner, ill 20 days, admitted Dec. 16th, 1841, with pain in the hepatic region, and diarrhœa; there was much tenderness below the margin of the right ribs, but the rest of the abdomen was supple, and not tender,—tongue dryish,—pulse 92—skin dry. By degrees he lost strength, and had occasional evening febrile accessions. He died Dec. 22d.

Autopsy.—Liver much enlarged, hard, friable, with much hypertrophy of its yellow tissue; (cirrhosis;) adhesions between the right lobe and the diaphragm; beneath this was a large abscess, occupying nearly the right lobe; it was not lined with any membrane, but had an uneven ragged surface; gall-bladder, small and flaccid, spleen small and hard, kidneys, and pancreas healthy; the colon, cæcum, and the lower part of the ilium extensively ulcerated. Externally, the body was yellow and emaciated, and the ribs of the right side were more prominent than those of the left. (*Dr. Morehead*, ibid, vol. vii, *p.* 49.)

No. 102.—T. Rich, sailor, æt. 22, ill 5 months, first with fever, followed by bowel complaint and pain in the right side; and, subsequently, by a short cough, with scanty expectoration; admitted March 22d, 1842. He was emaciated, the abdomen moderately distended, but without distinct enlargement of either the spleen or liver; bowels relaxed, skin warm, pulse frequent and feeble, tongue florid, cough troublesome, feet œdematous; the stools were pale and yeasty. On the 28th, he commenced expectorating purulent matter, and, under this combined with diarrhœa, he gradually sunk, and died May 1st.

Autopsy.—Liver enlarged; in the upper part of the right lobe was a large abscess, containing sero-purulent matter; it adhered to the diaphragm, as did the base of the right lung, and at this point the abscess communicated with the lung; other thoracic viscera healthy; the stomach and intestines attenuated. (*Dr. Morehead*, ibid, *p*. 50.)

No. 103.—C. Gordon, sailor, æt. 32, of very dissipated habits, subject to hepatitis, admitted Jan. 22d, 1843, with remittent fever. On the 30th, he began to complain of pain in the right side, attended with hard cough and irritability of the stomach; he was brought slightly under the influence of mercury. Till March 16th, he suffered chiefly from accessions of fever and debility; he then complained of increased pain in the hepatic region stretching to the shoulder, attended with short hacking cough, and sallow countenance. On the 27th, he expectorated much puriform matter, which continued till his death, May 17th.

Autopsy.—Purulent effusion in the right thoracic cavity; the lowest lobe of the right lung adhered firmly to the diaphragm, and on the opposed side of that muscle, the liver was also firmly adherent; at this point, in the substance of the liver, and quite superficial, was an abscess containing one pound of thick pus, having firm walls, but no distinct communication with the lung; the latter was slightly infiltrated with sero-purulent fluid, but crepitating; the liver dark-coloured and enlarged, but without any other abscess. (*Dr. Morehead*, ibid, vol. vii, *p*. 52.)

No. 104.—R. Carreth, sailor, æt. 25, admitted Feb. 22d, 1843, with hepatitis. The principal symptoms were occasional pain, never acute, in the right side, latterly some fulness at the epigastrium, and below the right ribs; also some tenseness, occasional vomiting, emaciation, loss of strength, night sweats, and diarrhœa—countenance pale. On June 1st, he was seized with cough and dyspnæa, and expectorated much purulent matter with a brick-red tinge. He died June 18th. Treatment. Leeches, sinapisms, quinine, camphor, and anodynes.

Autopsy.—Liver adherent to the diaphragm and right side; in the right lobe was an abscess, the size of an ostrich egg, filled with thick pus: its surface was flocculent, and a thin layer of condensed hepatic parenchyma formed the external walls; the lower part of the right lung hepatized; no distinct communication between the abscess and the lung was discovered, but the walls were readily lacerable, and the examination was not minute; lymph effused here and there on the surface of the intestines. (*Dr. Morehead*, ibid, vol. vii, *p*. 53.)

No. 105.—Sarah Corbin, æt. 32, admitted March 3rd, 1844. A week previously she fell on the edge of a tub, and hurt her side; and she complained of pain under the right mamma, augmented by full inspiration; leeches were applied. On the 5th, there was a febrile accession, with increase of pain in the side; and during the night she had profuse cold perspiration; on the 10th, there was irritability of the stomach. From this date she was easy, and left the hospital on the 18th, but was re-admitted on the 25th, with much pain in the right side, and a large, defined, tender tumour at the epigastrium. There was much nausea and vomiting, but no diarrhœa; skin coldish, pulse very feeble, breathing hurried. She died, April 13th.

Autopsy.—Two abscesses, one the size of an ostrich egg, on the concave part of the left lobe of the liver, immediately under the peritoneal covering; and another of nearly equal size, and also superficial, in the anterior part of the right lobe of the liver, and protected completely by the ribs. (*Dr. Morehead,* ibid, vol. vii, *p.* 54.)

No. 106.—J. Oakhum, æt. 32, feeble, emaciated, ill 8 days, admitted Sept. 27th, 1843, with pain of the right side, first under the clavicle, and subsequently at the margin of the right ribs; for this he was leeched and blistered. The principal symptoms were a marked evening febrile accession, and diarrhœa, but little pain in the side till Oct. 3d, when he was seized with cough, and expectoration of thin puriform fluid. There were afterwards febrile symptoms, dulness on percussion of the right side, occasional diarrhœa, emaciation, and collapse, and latterly, short and oppressed breathing. He died Oct. 12th.

Autopsy.—The right lung adherent to the diaphragm and ribs; in the pleural cavity were about 2 pounds of reddish-coloured puriform fluid; this effusion communicated through the diaphragm, with an abscess in the upper and posterior part of the right lobe of the liver, the size of a closed fist. The lung was compressed but healthy in structure; the intestines healthy externally. (*Dr. Morehead,* ibid, vol. vii, *p.* 54.)

No. 107.—J. Wilkinson, sailor, æt. 21, twice before treated for a cardiac affection with ascites; admitted, after drinking freely, Jan. 3d, 1841, with dysentery. There was fulness over the caput cæcum, and latterly much pain in the right hypochondrium. He gradually lost ground, and died January 24th.

Autopsy.—The liver, chiefly the right lobe, much enlarged, extending 4 inches below the ribs, and pushing the colon, almost into the hypogastrium; it was much congested, and here and there were abscesses, each the size of a walnut, with dark serous contents; some were quite superficial. Cæcum and colon ulcerated throughout—the left kidney enlarged—the right lung collapsed, but adherent to the diaphragm. The outer surface of the heart more pearly than natural, otherwise healthy.—(*Dr. Morehead*, ibid, vol. vii, *p*. 56.)

No. 108.—J. Greenwood, æt. 25, ill ten days with dysentery, admitted Dec. 11th, 1839. On the 20th evening, febrile exacerbations set in, and these continued more or less, with relaxed bowels, till his death, January 21st.

Autopsy.—In the right lobe of the liver were two abscesses, one the size of an orange, the other of a pigeon's egg; the walls of the former were flocculent, evidently the broken down parenchyma of the liver; the rest of the substance was mottled white and red. In the large intestines were some ulcers in the process of cicatrization. (*Dr. Morehead*, ibid, vol. vii, *p*. 57.)

No. 109.—C. Mitchell, æt. 24, 3 years in India, stout made, ill 13 days, admitted Dec. 13th, with dysentery. There was much uneasiness of the abdomen with tenesmus, and the stools contained much blood mixed with mucus or serum. He died January 3rd.

Autopsy.—Two abscesses in the liver, one, the size of an orange, in the right lobe, and another, the size of a walnut, in the left lobe. The large intestines thickened, and there were large patches of sloughy ulceration of the mucous surface, fringed with a layer of granular lymph. (*Dr. Morehead*, ibid, *p*. 57.)

No. 110.—H. Cassidy, æt. 25, ill 11 days, admitted Nov. 27th, 1840, with dysentery. The symptoms were acute, and were to a certain extent subdued, but the bowels continued relaxed, and there were occasional febrile accessions and loss of flesh. Subsequently, he had rigors, but no very marked fulness of the side. He became much emaciated, and died January 28th.

Autopsy.—Liver completely occupied the epigastric region; there were two abscesses; one in the centre of the right lobe, the other in the left lobe; colon contracted, and presented numerous ulcerations, some of them cicatrizing. Incipient yellow degeneration of both kidneys—mesenteric glands enlarged—stomach healthy—lungs collapsed, but healthy. On the surface of the heart were some pearly opaque patches. (*Dr. Morehead*, vol. vii, *p*. 57.)

No. 111.—J. Harrison, sailor, æt. 55, ill 4 days, admitted July 14th, with dysentery. The symptoms were never very urgent, but they were never completely subdued. He progressively lost flesh and strength, and never complained of pain in the right side. There was no palpable enlargement any where in the abdomen. He died September 10th.

Autopsy.—In the right lobe of the liver was an abscess containing 12 oz. of pus. Throughout the large intestines were numerous transverse ulcers, some sloughing, others cicatrizing; the end of the ilium was healthy; there was great displacement of the colon, such as is not unfrequently seen in dysenteric cases. Stomach and kidneys healthy—lungs collapsed. (*Dr. Morehead*, ibid, vol. vii, *p.* 58.)

No. 112.—J. Slayman, sailor, æt. 32, admitted August 20th, with dysentery; abdomen tender, pulse full, skin and tongue dry. On the 22d, there was tenderness of the right iliac region, with perceptible hardness. There was also much tenesmus, a moderately distended abdomen, more or less dysuria, and the stools were brown and watery, with dysenteric fetor—he also passed patches of sloughed mucous membrane. He died Sept. 10th, 1840. Treatment. Depletion, local and general; blue pill and ipecacuanha, opium, acetate of lead, &c.

Autopsy.—Liver enlarged, extending into the left hypochondrium; in the right lobe, about half an inch from the surface, was an abscess the size of an orange; large intestines extensively ulcerated, the mucous coat in parts separated and thrown off; the lower end of the ilium healthy; colon much displaced; pyloric extremity of the stomach mammillated; kidneys healthy. (*Dr. Morehead*, ibid, vol. vii, *p.* 59.)

No. 113.—J. Higgs, æt. 21, recently from England, ill 5 days; admitted Dec. 10th, 1839, with dysentery. He was freely bled and took mercury, but was not brought under its influence; the dysenteric symptoms were sometimes better, at others worse; then febrile accessions with remissions set in, and he died Jan. 30th.

Autopsy.—There was a circumscribed purulent sac between the liver and the concavity of the right false ribs; also two abscesses in the right lobe, near the diaphragm; the large intestines ulcerated throughout. (*Dr. Morehead*, ibid, vol. vii.)

No. 114.—E. Clarke, sailor, æt. 24, slight made, dark complexion, under treatment for rheumatism from May 26th to 31st, discharged well; re-admitted June 6th, with dysentery. There was much fulness and pain in the abdomen, with tenesmus; countenance anxious; pulse frequent, feeble; tongue white; stools yellow, slimy, and streaked with blood; the abdomen remained full and tense, but the other symptoms were chiefly those of acute dysentery. He died on the 19th, having been comatose about half an hour. There was vomiting the day before death.

Autopsy.—Liver pale in texture; in the left lobe was an abscess the size of a walnut; large intestines in a state of sloughy ulceration; mucous coat of the stomach mammillated; mesenteric glands enlarged; kidneys healthy; lungs emphysematous; effusion of 2 ounces of serum at the base of the skull. (*Dr. Morehead*, ibid, vol. vii.)

No. 115.—C. Moriarty, æt. 45, of dissipated habits; after drinking to excess, admitted Nov. 7th, 1840, with tenderness in the right iliac region; the abdomen was tender, pulse feeble, tongue florid, hands tremulous. The subsequent history of the case was obscure, from the supervention of delirium tremens and dysentery. The chief symptoms were tenderness at the margin of the right ribs, nausea and vomiting, with a tongue florid at the edges and tip, and coated in the centre. He died on the 11th.

Autopsy.—Liver enlarged, brittle, and hard, containing 7 or 8 small abscesses, the largest of the size of a walnut, and the others, the size of horse-beans; the smaller ones were filled with thick adhesive pus, and the larger ones had the appearance of the parenchyma infiltrated with purulent matter, not yet broken down. Sloughy ulcerations in the colon, and two in the rectum. (*Dr. Morehead*, ibid, *p.* 65.)

No. 116.—E. Burnard, sailor, æt. 58, ill 15 days; admitted Sept. 25th, with diarrhœa and occasional vomiting. On the 26th, there was tenderness along the right side, from the crest of the ilium to the margin of the ribs; the stools copious, frequent, yellow, with some mucus and blood. Subsequently there was pain on pressure in the right hypochondrium; tongue without fur, pusle 92 feeble; skin moist and coldish, countenance anxious, breathing hurried. He died Oct. 3d.

Autopsy.—Extensive peritonitis; convolutions of the intestines and the omentum, matted together; on separating these adhesions, several patched up ulcerations gave way, and the contents of the large intestines escaped; the coats readily friable; in the convex surface of the right lobe of the liver was one abscess, the size of a walnut. (*Dr. Morehead*, ibid, vol. vii, *p.* 72.)

No. 117.—D. Donahen, æt. 28, stout made, dissipated, ill 12 days; admitted Dec. 11th, 1842, with dysentery; there was much tenderness about the cæcum, heat of skin, and frequent pulse; he was bled, and took a full dose of calomel and opium. On the 14th, he was delirious, and there was distinct hardness over the cæcum; opiates were given freely, but the dysenteric symptoms were unabated, and on the 29th, there was uneasiness of the right side, extending to the shoulder. Occasional febrile symptoms, collapsing features, and declining strength preceded his death, Jan. 4th, 1843.

Autopsy.—Adhesions between the omentum, the cæcum, and the colon; the liver, in a state of cirrhosis, with several small abscesses projecting from its convex surface; there was a larger one, at the thin edge of the liver, the walls of which were in part formed by the omentum. (*Dr. Morehead,* ibid, vol. vii, *p.* 76.)

No. 118.—S. Duran, æt. 29, sailor, ill 4 days with dysentery; admitted July 29th, 1843. Under the use of leeches, blue pill, ipecacuanha, &c., the symptoms improved, and on Aug. 6th, the report is, "the frequency of purging decreased much, the stools yellow, feculent and more copious, the abdomen supple, the skin, pulse, and tongue improved." He continued improving till Aug. 11th, when evening febrile accessions, with sweating during the night commenced, and continued daily, with increasing severity. There was no pain of the abdomen complained of, but the fulness returned; the stools were feculent till the 22d, when they again became tinged with blood. He died Aug. 24th.

Autopsy.—Liver enlarged, reaching 3 inches below the margin of the ribs; deep-seated in the right lobe was a large abscess, with thickened walls, containing one pound of thick pus; the mucous coat of the colon and cæcum was of a dark-grey colour, with many large circular ulcers, all showing more or less a tendency to cicatrize; the contents of the colon consisted of thin feculence. (*Dr. Morehead,* ibid, vol. vii, *p.* 78.)

No. 119.—W. Spence, sailor, æt. 43, ill a month with fever and dysentery, admitted Oct. 5th, 1843. He had much purging, a sense of weight and uneasiness of the right side, and some tension at the margin of the right ribs. He continued affected with frequent purging, occasional uneasiness across the chest, but without any distinct fulness of the right side; frequently an evening febrile accession, and latterly much vomiting and emaciation; the tongue was slightly coated at the centre, but not florid at the tip or edges; pulse feeble. He died Oct. 22d. Opiates constituted the chief remedy.

Autopsy.—Liver enlarged; in the centre of the right lobe was an abscess, the size of a hen's egg, with a thin membranous lining; the colon presented a dark-brown, in parts, a black irregular aspect (melanosis) with ulcers, some circular and others longitudinal; the inner surface of the cæcum was also in a black sloughy state; mesenteric glands enlarged. (*Dr. Morehead,* ibid, vol. vii, *p.* 79.)

No. 120.—M. Quiley, æt. 25, 19½ years in India, an Irishman, admitted with dysentery, Nov. 18th, and died November 27th, 1840; duration of the disease 22 days. History of the case not given.

Autopsy.—General peritonitis; the large intestines bound to contiguous parts by lymph; abscesses in their walls; mucous coat already separated, or in sloughy patches; invagination of the lower end of the transverse colon; liver with corrugated surface, and two abscesses in the right lobe. (*Dr. Leith, Trans. of Med. and Phys. Society of Bombay*, vol. iv, *p.* 74.)

No. 121.—W. Griggs, æt. 36, Englishman, 19½ years in India, admitted with dysentery, Nov. 18th, and died Nov. 27th, 1840; duration of the disease 14 days. History of the case not given.

Autopsy.—Liver enlarged, adherent to the diaphragm; two abscesses in the left lobe, and two in the right; substance degenerated, speckled yellow and red; mucous membrane of the large intestines inflamed, sloughy or separated; cæcum and colon a mass of disease, with abscesses in their walls; a nearly cartilaginous ring at each end of the transverse arch. (*Dr. Leith,* ibid, vol. x, *p.* 74.)

No. 122.—J. Cottis, æt. 21, 2 years in India, slender, of melancholic temperament, admitted May 8th, 1842, with remittent fever attended by nausea and acute catching pain at the epigastrium, checking his breathing. Under V. S., leeches, blue pill, opium, &c., the pain was relieved, and on the 19th, the report is, "Feels quite easy, only weak; skin pretty cool; tongue covered with a dark moist load; bowels active; pulse 96; hepatic dulness from the nipple to an inch in front of the cartilaginous border, and from the apex of the right scapula downwards, with crepitating râles, over all the subscapular region, and round superiorly to the nipple. On the 28th, the abdomen was tense and semi-tympanitic, and blue superficial veins were observed meandering over the right hypochondrium. He died June 5th.

Autopsy.—The right lobe of the liver, and the lower portion of the right lung were occupied by an immense abscess filled with thin greenish matter; it was lined with a cyst, and no traces of vessels were observable, except two or three short fleshy shreds; the lower lobe of the lung was completely removed, ulcerated off horizontally; and laterally the pleura, adhering to the ribs, formed part of the sac; the cæcal valve and six inches of the colon, closely set with large circular ulcers, having thickened edges; left lobe of the liver straw-coloured. (*R. H. Hunter, Esq. Trans. of Med. and Phys. Society of Bombay*, vol. v, *p.* 52.)

No. 123.—R. McGuffie, æt. 40, ill a month; admitted Dec. 30th, 1846, with dysentery. There was no abdominal tenderness, even on the closest pressure; the evacuations were frequent, and consisted of dark-coloured serum, more or less mixed with grumous blood. He took calomel, opium, ipecacuanha, &c., but no improvement ensued, and he died Jan. 6th.

Autopsy.—Liver much enlarged, with an abscess containing 8 oz. of pus in the upper portion of the right lobe; extensive ulceration in the colon, which in parts was softened and sphacelated. (*Dr. M. Stovell, Tr. of Med. & Phys. Society of Bombay*, vol. ix, *p.* 56.)

No. 124.—G. Wood, æt. 37, recently from England, admitted Dec. 31st, 1846, with dysentery. There was frequent purging of slime and blood, tenesmus, pain in the course of the ascending colon, and great heat of skin; pulse rapid; tongue thickly furred. He was leeched and took calomel, opium, and ipecacuanha, but with little benefit. He died Jan. 11th.

Autopsy.—Liver greatly enlarged and softened, with three abscesses in the right lobe, and one in the left; mucous membrane of the small intestines of an ashy appearance; that of the large intestines ulcerated, though not to a great extent; a tubular portion of the mucous coat was found depending from the anus. (*Dr. M. Stovell,* ibid, vol. ix, *p.* 57.)

No. 125.—G. Rigby, æt. 47, admitted July 3d, 1846; ill 8 days with dysentery. There was frequent purging of slime and blood, with an occasional trace of feculence; no abdominal tenderness. Severe dyspnæa supervened on the 18th, and he died next day, the 19th.

Autopsy.—Three abscesses in the liver, two in the right, and one in the left lobe, containing altogether about two pounds of healthy pus; liver and the right lung adherent to the opposed sides of the diaphragm, and a small quantity of pus had made its way from the abscess into the bronchi; in the colon were a few patches of ulceration. (*Dr. M. Stovell,* ibid, *p.* 58.)

No. 126.—Ellen Watten, æt. 37; 8 months in India, admitted Sept. 3d, 1846, with acute hepatitis; the pain in the hepatic region was severe, increased by pressure and full inspiration; bowels very irritable, pulse 100. Under the use of leeches, calomel and opium, blisters, &c., she much improved; the pain quite subsided, and she had no night sweats, nor febrile accessions; pulse falling to 88, and becoming quite soft. Subsequently the bowels became again relaxed, and on Oct. 1st, she was seized with severe vomiting and purging, the stools not containing any purulent matter. She died Oct. 6th.

Autopsy.—Liver greatly enlarged, extending into the left hypochondrium and below the umbilicus; in the right lobe was a large abscess containing two pounds of pus. Other viscera healthy. (*Dr. Stovell,* ibid, vol. ix, *p.* 61.)

No. 127.—R. Black, æt. 29, bilious temperament, ill some days with diarrhœa, but without abdominal tenderness; admitted Dec. 18th, 1846,—he had severe pain in the liver, not increased by pressure, but much augmented by taking a full inspiration, and by lying on the back or left side. Under the use of leeches, blisters, calomel, &c., the pain subsided, but the bowels became irritable, and he began to sweat profusely at nights. He gradually wasted away, and died Jan. 17th.

Autopsy.—Liver congested, but of normal size; in the upper and posterior part of the right lobe was an abscess containing two pounds of pus. Other viscera healthy. (*Dr. Stovell,* ibid, vol. ix, *p.* 61.)

No. 128.—C. Craggs, sailor, æt. 17, delicate, of light complexion, one month in India, ill 14 days—admitted June 24th, 1830, with dysentery; there was slight fulness across the epigastrium, very little pyrexia, pulse 100; under the use of V. S., leeches, blisters, calomel, and purgatives, the enlargement of the liver appeared reduced, the tumefaction varying from day to day, sometimes hardly perceptible, but the abdominal muscles remained tense. He became weak, languid, fretful, and desponding; pulse rapid; stools frequent and watery, sometimes tinged with blood, often nearly dark. He died July 13th. There were no rigors at any period of the disease.

Autopsy.—Liver enlarged, adhesion between the convex surface of the right lobe and the diaphragm; under this was a large abscess, containing 2 pounds of matter, mostly puriform, the rest a brownish serum. Left lobe adherent to the stomach; in it was an abscess containing 5 oz. of glutinous brown thick fluid; its walls were in a sloughing state; the gall-bladder shrunk and flaccid, contained a little opaque, orange-coloured, oily fluid. In the colon were numerous small ulcerations; the mucous coat of the rectum vascular, and somewhat abraded; right lung adherent to the diaphragm. (*Twining, Diseases of Bengal, 2d Ed.*, vol. i, *p.*311.)

No. 129.—H. King, sailor, æt. 24, 2 years in India, in hospital with continued fever, discharged well May 13th, 1830; indulged freely in spirits; re-admitted June 14th, with enlarged liver, and pyrexia, pulse 112. He was bled, and took calomel and purgatives, but he became weak and fretful, the liver remaining large, and he died June 25th. He had no rigors or dysenteric symptoms.

Autopsy.—Liver much enlarged; the convex surface of the right lobe adhered to the diaphragm; at this point was a large abscess extending into the centre of the liver; gall-bladder flaccid, covered with a false membrane, adherent to the colon; right lung adherent to the diaphragm. (*Twining*, ibid, vol. i, *p*. 314.)

No. 130.—G. N., sailor, æt. 27, stout, tall, muscular, of light complexion, lately from England, was attacked Jan. 23d, 1838, with fever, tenseness and fulness at the epigastrium, and pain over the whole of the right side of the chest and abdomen. He was actively treated, and took calomel in large and repeated doses, with the view of inducing ptyalism, but without effect. The pain was relieved but not removed, the pulse remained full, the skin dry, and the tongue much loaded with mucus. On Feb. 10th, he had a troublesome cough, with copious puriform expectoration of a yellow bilious hue and bitter taste. This continued till his death, Feb. 28th.

Autopsy.—An enormous abscess of the right lobe of the liver was found to have opened into the right lung, which was adherent to the upper surface of the diaphragm, and was in a state of induration and suppuration. The state of the intestines not given. (*Twining*, ibid, vol. i, *p*. 315.)

No. 131.—D. Dominique, a French sailor, æt. 44, dark complexioned, steady, temperate, ill 8 days, admitted Dec. 4th, 1830, with hepatitis; he was pale and much exhausted, abdomen tense, liver very hard, had a troublesome cough, pulse weak, tongue white, bowels costive. Under the use of leeches, purgatives, calomel, &c., he much improved, but after indulging in a quantity of improper food, a relapse ensued; the cough returned, followed by emaciation, a peculiar sharpness of visage, and dysenteric symptoms. He then lost all hope, refused to take any remedies, the stools became dark-brown, watery, mixed with blood, and of a putrid odour. The pulse did not exceed 86 when in a recumbent posture. He died Jan. 8th.

Autopsy.—Liver enlarged, indurated, of a pale drab color, the convex surface of the right lobe adherent to the space between the 7th and 8th ribs, and at this part contained a large abscess, very near the surface; the margin of the right lobe adherent to the colon. Numerous small ulcers in the colon and rectum; mesenteric glands enlarged; universal adhesions of the right lung. (*Twining*, ibid, vol. i, *p*. 318.)

No. 132.—Hollman, æt. 37, 18 years in India, a very sober temperate man, of abstemious habits, spare frame, middle size, light complexion, was seized on Oct. 9th, with "cold and headache." Under the use of leeches and purgatives he was soon better, but on the 16th, he had a return of fever preceded by chilliness, (but no rigor,) pulse 62, rather hard. He remained never entirely free from fever, but with a distinct exacerbation every evening; the stools were frequent, scanty, and dark coloured; there was elastic tension of the epigastrium, and some dyspnæa, but no pain in the shoulder; tongue loaded with thick white mucus. 18th, "Urine high coloured, cough, anxiety, obliged to rest with his head and shoulders much raised, flatulent eructations, no pain or pressure over the liver, tension at the epigastrium continues." 20th, "Pulse 104, fever not very strong, the evening exacerbations less distinct, stools frequent, copious, dark brown, watery—no pain, but flatulence and tension of the epigastrium. Mouth affected by mercury, the gums red and painful, but without free ptyalism." Nov. 1st, "Tongue loaded in the centre with brownish mucus, the edges of a morbid red." These symptoms continued more or less till his death, Nov. 12th.

Autopsy.—Liver enlarged, its convex surface covered with a thick coat of coagulable lymph, and it contained two large deep-seated abscesses; the left lobe adhered to the stomach, the right to the colon. In this viscus were numerous small circular ulcers. (*Twining*, ibid, *p.* 321.)

No. 133.—J. Thompson, sailor, æt. 50, 9 months in the Indian seas, slight made, of dark complexion, admitted Sept. 20th, 1830, with enlarged liver, for which he had been treated on board ship for 14 days. When admitted, his mouth was sore from mercury, the liver enormously large, so as to be seen as well as felt below the cartilages of the ribs. He had no pyrexia, no pain in the shoulder, the pulse 84, soft, rather full, and it did not exceed 86 until the day when the abscess burst. He was depleted locally and generally, and took calomel and purgatives, but without decreasing the enlargement of the liver. On the 29th of Sept., at 10 P. M., he became very uneasy and agitated, the pulse rose to 124, he was incoherent, the feet became cold, and the tumefaction of the liver subsided. He was restless all night, and died at 3 A. M.

Autopsy.—Liver enormously enlarged, dark, soft, easily torn, a large abscess at the lower edge of the right lobe had burst into the cavity of the abdomen—no adhesions to contiguous parts. There were ulcerations in the cæcum, and some old adhesions in both lungs. (*Twining*, vol. i, *p.* 331.)

No. 134.—J. Backhofen, æt. 44, a small pale man, admitted July 19th, 1833, with tumefaction and hardness at the epigastrium, and pressure caused acute pain; respiration impeded, pulse

84, soft, and weak, feet swollen; has been ill for some months. Leeches, blisters, blue pill, and purgatives employed. On the 23d, he was suddenly seized with a violent pain in the abdomen, attended with anxiety, a rapid, weak pulse, prostration of strength, and cold extremities. The skin and eyes became yellow, and the evacuations by stools and urine were for a time suppressed. Subsequently, diarrhœa supervened, and he died Aug. 18th, 26 days after the abscess apparently burst into the abdomen.

Autopsy.—Liver and omentum universally adherent to the adjacent parts, and an enormous abscess in the former had burst into the cavity of the peritoneum. (*Twining*, ibid, vol. i, *p.* 333.)

No. 135.—J. Painter, æt. 39, Indo-Briton, admitted May 15th, 1833, much emaciated, ill for a month with purging. The liver was enlarged, the abdominal muscles tense, abdomen flat and inelastic, tongue dry, nearly clean, pulse from 104 to 110. Depletion, blisters, and mild mercurials employed. May 22d, emaciation gradually increased, had occasionally pain in the right shoulder, and constant diarrhœa. June 9th, felt a sudden pain shooting from the region of the liver down to the lower part of the abdomen; the pulse immediately rose to 126, and he suffered much from anxiety, coldness, and debility; the abdomen became exquisitely painful on the slightest pressure. On the 15th, he had some dysuria, and he died on the following day.

Autopsy.—Liver enlarged and softened, adherent to the diaphragm; in the lower and outer portion of the right lobe was a large abscess, which had opened into the cavity of the abdomen, and about 5 ounces of pus had flowed down into the pelvis. A large quantity of thick and nearly white pus remained in the abscess, the sides of which were covered with a thick, hard, white lining, which was rough on account of numerous small projecting eminences; the peritoneum inflamed; mesenteric glands enlarged. (*Twining*, ibid, *p.* 336.)

No. 136.—J. Sticklie, æt. 48, sailor, tall, thin, of light complexion, admitted Jan. 25th, 1829, having been long ill with enlarged liver and dysentery. He had been bled and blistered, and had taken mercury to the extent of slightly affecting his mouth, before admission. He was then weak and exhausted, had a dry brown tongue, general tenseness of the abdomen, and enlargement of the liver; pulse 116. He died Jan. 27th.

Autopsy.—Liver large and slightly mottled on the surface; it contained five distinct abscesses, two large and deep-seated, in the centre of the right lobe; one small one near the anterior edge, and two others, not half the size of a marble, just below the surface, at the convex portion of the same lobe, but evident through the peritoneal coat. On the concave surface of the left lobe was a distinct ecchymosed spot, the size of a small bean; the colon was contracted, and in the transverse portion were a few small circular ulcers, and cicatrices of others. Mr. Twining observes that this is the only case in which he met with the whole series of the disease, consisting of ecchymosis, small abscesses, and large abscesses, in the same subject; the lungs presented old adhesions, but were otherwise healthy. (*Twining*, ibid, vol. i, *p*. 337.)

No. 137.—Lowder, 2 years in India, admitted Sept. 22d, 1831, in the lowest state of misery and distress, having been ill with purging for 9 weeks. On admission he had frequent calls to stool, and voided much blood, part of which was in coagula; pulse 124, weak, hands cold, occasional hiccough; he was unable to lie on either side, but was obliged to rest on his back, with his shoulders a little raised; there was fulness at the epigastrium inclining somewhat to the right side, but the rest of the abdomen was flat and inelastic; pressure caused little pain, except at the epigastrium. He continued cold and low, and died Sept. 27th.

Autopsy.—The liver was rather larger and paler than usual, and there was an abscess under the ligamentum latum, the size of half an orange; there were slight soft adhesions for the space of ¾ths of an inch round the abscess; the walls were in a sloughing state, and the diaphragm only interfered between the upper edge of the sac and the pericardium; in the colon were numerous sloughing ulcers; the gall-bladder was covered with a false membrane, and was rather smaller than natural. (*Twining*, ibid, vol. i, *p*. 338.)

No. 138.—J. Iuden, æt. 33, had been under treatment for hepatitis, and was discharged apparently well; the next day he was seized with cold shivering, succeeded by heat, abdominal pain, and vomiting. Re-admitted April 26th, 1816. The principal symptoms were vomiting, great sense of heat at the pit of the stomach, with much flatulence, and frequent eructations of acrid air; the stools were at first clay-coloured, and afterwards dark-green, liquid, and offensive; the pulse 96, soft, latterly irritable; much depression of spirits, thirst, restlessness, and impaired appetite. Purgatives, calomel, salines, &c., were given with little benefit. On May 6th, an obscure tumour was detected under the right false ribs; he had hitherto had no pain in the abdomen, (except flatulence,) and none now except on pressure being made; next day he passed by stool about 3 pounds of pus and coagula of blood, by which he felt much weakened; the tumour at the side subsided at the same time. He died on the 10th Instant.

Autopsy.—In the right lobe of the liver was a large abscess containing a mixture of grumous blood and pus; it was situated on the concave surface, and was found to have burst into the colon; this intestine was much contracted, and contained numerous small ulcerations; the small intestines, stomach, spleen and thoracic viscera healthy. (*Annesley, Diseases of India, 4to Ed.*, vol. i, *p.* 518.)

No. 139.—W. Bedlow, admitted with hepatitis; was actively treated by depletion, mercurials, purgatives, and salines for two months, but without any permanent benefit. It appears to have been a purely chronic case; the pulse was soft, ranging from 66 to 84, but never exceeding the latter number; the tongue was at first foul, but latterly became perfectly clean and natural; skin normal, appetite indifferent, rest disturbed; he had great oppression on the chest, much pain in the liver, increased on pressure, or by lying on the right side. No fluctuation was detected, neither does the disease appear to have been complicated with any other affection. The stools were quite feculent, till within a few days of death; there was general soreness throughout the abdomen, but there was no distinct or evident swelling of the side; on pressure, however, over the liver, there was pain which he described as shooting through the shoulder and the collar bone. Two days before death, Jan, 15th, the stools were perfectly natural.

Autopsy.—The liver was much enlarged, descending into the right iliac region, and filling the whole of the epigastrium and the right and left hypochondriac regions; there were two abscesses, one on the concave surface of each lobe, containing well digested pus; there was much displacement of the stomach and large intestines, the coats of the latter being much thickened and contracted—in places much thinned, but without any ulceration. (*Annesley*, ibid, vol. i, *p.* 535.)

No. 140.—P. Hurd, had been treated for dysentery, and under the use of remedies including mercurials, he was convalescent, when symptoms of hepatic derangement manifested themselves. On the 18th, it is reported for the first time, pain over the whole abdomen on pressure, particularly in the right and left sides, in the course of the colon, and about the umbilicus; there was no fulness nor tension complained of, and no pain except on pressure; the pulse was small, quick, and trembling; the tongue furred, brown, and dry. Latterly there was vomiting of green bilious matter like verdigris; the stools were reported as feculent on the day prior to death, Jan. 21st.

Autopsy.—The liver much enlarged; there was one abscess on the convex surface of the right lobe, firmly adherent to the diaphragm, and another small abscess in the left lobe; gall-bladder very small, and its coats much thickened; there was much displacement of the intestines, but their mucous coat presented no marked appearance of disease; the pancreas, together with the duodenum, gall-bladder and contiguous parts were matted together. (*Annesley*, ibid, vol. i, *p*. 539.)

No. 141.—Lieut. ——, H. M. 59th Regt., reported sick Dec. 17th, 1815, at Calcutta. He had constant vomiting, and his system could not be brought under the influence of mercury; previously he had pain in the side extending to the shoulder and across the abdomen, but it was relieved by leeches and other remedies. Emesis took place without exertion, and the fluids were ejected nearly unchanged; occasionally a good deal of green watery fluid was thrown up. He had for some time an undefined swelling below the pit of the stomach, together with cough and pain in the side and chest, augmented by change of position; reclining on the back was the easiest posture; he was also troubled with hiccup; the bowels were open, latterly "out of order;" the pulse and skin almost natural. He was delirious for two days before death, on Dec. 26th.

Autopsy.—The liver was very large, adherent to contiguous parts, and also very firmly to the right side from the 5th rib to the lower false ribs, and pressing on the diaphragm; the right lobe was one immense abscess, containing greenish and liverish-coloured matter; in the left lobe were many small vomica, and a kind of cheesy tubercle; there was ulceration of the large intestines; gall-bladder distended with ropy green bile; the heart was large, and the pericardium contained a large quantity of blackish fluid. (*Annesley*, ibid, vol. i, *p*. 541.)

No. 142.—R. Morris, long ill, admitted Dec. 27th, with oppression on the chest, cough, with copious and bloody expectoration, and inability to lie on his back from a sense of suffocation; he had no particular pain in his side, the bowels regular, stools natural, pulse 120. Local depletion, anodynes, and demulcents were employed without benefit; he died Jan. 2d, six days after admission.

Autopsy.—The liver was enormously enlarged, filling the whole of the right and left hypochondriac, the epigastric and a great part of the umbilical region; in the superior convex part was an immense abscess, which communicated with another large abscess in the right lung; it contained between 3 and 4 quarts of pus. The substance of the liver was tender and soft, and the abscess walls were ulcerated, and tore on the slightest pressure; in the pericardium were 8 or 9 ounces of serum; the substance of the lungs softened, the mesenteric glands much enlarged, the large intestines much contracted, but without ulceration; gall-bladder full of yellow bile. (*Annesley*, ibid, vol. i, *p.* 542.)

No. 143.—J. Lynch, æt. 27, admitted June 4th, with constipation and pain in the bowels of some days standing; this was soon followed by pain in the right side, great thirst, and much anxiety. Under the use of leeches, mercurial purgatives, and salines, these symptoms partially subsided, but he was much troubled with flatulence, and also with cough; pulse soft, from 84 to 90; skin moist and warm, tongue latterly of a peculiar smooth, shining appearance, which Annesley regards as a sign of organic disease of the liver; appetite good, and there was not much thirst, except after the exhibition of cinchona; the stools were feculent, natural, and scybalous. At no period does there appear to have been any fulness, or sensible enlargement of the side; neither pressure nor deep inspiration increased the hepatic pain, and the respiration was perfectly free. He died July 14th.

Autopsy.—The liver much enlarged; in the right lobe was an immense abscess, containing 3 quarts of white pus; the lower portion of the ilium somewhat ulcerated; the large intestines in a state of sloughing ulceration throughout; the coats of the colon were as thin as paper, but at its commencement at the cæcum, it was converted into a cartilaginous mass; lungs healthy, with the exception of some adhesions. (*Annesley*, ibid, vol. i, *p.* 544.)

No. 144.—J. Donelly, æt. 26, 5 months in India, admitted Dec. 17th, 1816, with dull heavy pain in the bowels, dysenteric purging, a bitter taste in the mouth, and vertigo; pulse quick and small, tongue white. The treatment consisted of leeches, blisters, calomel in large doses, and aperients. The symptoms of dysentery appear quite to have masked those of the hepatic abscess; indeed, cold sweats were almost the only ordinary symptom of the latter affection. At no period had he pain or tumefaction of the side, and no mention is made of rigors, vomiting, or cough; the stools, which were at first dysenteric, became black, watery, and offensive; and the tongue, from being white and dry, became perfectly clean and natural; there was much drowsiness and thirst, the skin was dry and cool, and the pulse feeble, ranging from 80 to 102. He died Jan. 4th.

Autopsy.—The liver much enlarged, filling the whole of the hypochondriac and epigastric regions, and extending into the right iliac region; in the upper and convex part of the right lobe an immense abscess formed a cyst, containing two quarts of pus. The large intestines were in a state of sloughing ulceration throughout, and through perforations in the coats, their contents had escaped into the abdominal cavity, causing general peritonitis and agglutination of the intestines; one large ulcer was found in the ilium. (*Annesley,* ibid, vol. i, *p.* 547.)

No. 145.—J. Collins, æt. 47, long in India, admitted Dec. 20th, 1820, with acute pain in the hepatic region, pain in the shoulder, and inability to lie on the left side; his gums were swollen and tender, mouth clammy, pulse 120, skin natural, tongue slightly white, countenance anxious and sallow, urine high coloured, appetite impaired. Subsequently he had cold sweats, a troublesome cough with expectoration of phlegm, pain chiefly at the posterior part of the liver, increased by pressure and inspiration, hurried and oppressed breathing, and much fulness and tenseness of the right side; the stools were dark, fetid and copious; pulse 120, small; much thirst, great exhaustion. Leeches, alterative doses of calomel, salines, and palliatives formed the main treatment.

Autopsy.—In the concave surface of the right lobe was a large abscess, which had apparently burst into the abdominal cavity shortly before death; much matter had escaped; the gall-bladder was filled with a greenish-brown fluid; there was general peritonitis, and the colon was in a state of ulceration; the right lung was adherent to the diaphragm. (*Annesley,* ibid, vol. i, *p.* 550.)

No. 146.—J. Glover, admitted April 1st, with hepatitis, which yielded to bleeding and purging; the mouth became nearly sore from mercury, and though the pain diminished, he became much reduced, and had frequent cold sweats; the pulse was irritable, and the stools morbid, and in the latter he passed some lumbrici; the subsequent symptoms were cold shiverings, much perspiration, nausea, and vomiting, much thirst and restlessness; the stools consisted of blood and slime, or were green, feculent, and viscid. He had pain in the side, described as teasing; latterly, however, this disappeared, and for the last three days of his life, he is stated to have been free from pain, He died April 5th.

Autopsy.—The liver enlarged; on its convex surface was a large abscess attached to the diaphragm, which formed part of its cyst; it contained watery curdled matter of various colours; near this, also on the convex surface, was another large abscess full of thick, white, well digested pus; the left lobe was of a leaden hue, but without any abscess; the gall-bladder was full of thick inspissated green bile; the ducts were amazingly dilated, their coats much thickened and hardened, almost cartilaginous; the small intestines inflated, empty, and transparent; in the cæcum and colon were ulcerations and traces of inflammation; the spleen, kidneys, hearts, and lungs presented nothing abnormal. (*Annesley*, ibid, vol. i, *p.* 552.)

No. 147.—Smith, a fine robust soldier, recently from England, admitted Aug. 13th, 1819, with symptoms of dysentery supervening on acute hepatitis; his pulse was full and strong, the dysenteric symptoms urgent; he also had pain in the side, with a troublesome cough; depletion, calomel, blisters, and salines were employed with little effect. Dyspnæa, with an urgent sense of suffocation and cough came on, and he died with all the signs of hydrothorax, on the 26th Instant.

Autopsy.—In the superior surface of the liver was an immense abscess, which had partly emptied itself into the right thoracic cavity, and partly into the bronchical ramifications of the right lung, through the diaphragm; upwards of a gallon of whey-like matter was collected altogether; the right lung was adherent to the diaphragm, at the point at which the abscess opened; but the adhesions had either been incomplete, or they had partially given way, at the time of the flow of the purulent matter into the thoracic cavity; the gall-bladder contained very little bile; the intestines were not materially diseased. (*Annesley*, ibid, vol. i, *p.* 558.)

No. 148.—C. Rymer, under treatment with chronic hepatitis, for which leeches had been applied, and blue pill and purgatives administered. Subsequently there was a dull heavy pain in the side, increased by deep inspiration; pain over the abdomen generally, and urgent thirst; the countenance was sallow, the skin cool, the pulse from 86 to 92, the appetite pretty good; the stools were feculent, dark, and frothy, and latterly they contained purulent matter; urine scanty and high coloured; mercurial frictions were employed, at the same time that the blue pill was continued internally. On the 24th of July, ascites having supervened, the operation of paracentesis abdominis was performed, and much fluid drawn off; immediately after the operation, the urine became clear, but distressing hiccup set in. On the 5th of August, the fluid having again accumulated, the operation was repeated; a quart of nearly pure water first came away, *the rest of the fluid withdrawn was mixed with about two pounds of healthy pus.* On Aug. 8th, the fluid having again accumulated, the operation was again performed, and on this occasion eight quarts of fluid mixed with healthy pus were removed. On the 16th, the operation was rendered necessary for the fourth time, and eight pints of fluid, nearly one-half of which was pus, were evacuated; the discharge of purulent matter from the orifice continued till the date of the patient's death, on the 24th Inst., being 19 days from the date at which matter began to be discharged.

Autopsy.—In the abdominal cavity were found about 6 pounds of serum and blood. The liver was enlarged and flaccid; in the right lobe was the cyst of an abscess containing a small quantity of pus and grumous blood; the point of rupture into the abdominal cavity was at the edge of the concave surface of the liver; in the colon and the rectum some slight ulcerations were found; stomach, spleen, and kidneys natural; the omentum was a thickened putrid mass, extending over and closely adhering to the surface of the intestines; the left lung a mass of suppuration; the right lung slightly affected. Effusion of 5 ounces of serum in the pericardium. (*Annesley*, ibid, vol. i, *p.* 559.)

No. 149.—M. Clinch, admitted Dec. 23d, 1814, with hepatitis of long standing. He had considerable tumefaction at the margin of the ribs, with much tenderness, purging, and a cold clammy state of the skin; his countenance was livid, pulse 96 and small, the tongue foul and dark, and encrusted with mucus; mercury, externally and internally, was used, together with salines, tonics, and latterly, cinchona. The pain in the side appears to have subsided, as on the 26th, it is recorded that there was no pain or complaint on pressure of the abdomen; the tongue also much improved, being on the 27th, (the day before death,) moist and clean; pulse 89 to 90, regular, soft, and small; the stools consisted of blood and mucus, and latterly contained purulent matter; there were cold sweats, especially of the extremities, but no rigors. He was delirious for two days prior to death on the 28th Instant.

Autopsy.—The liver was enlarged and a mass of disease; it contained three large distinct abscesses; one had burst into the arch of the colon, to which it was adherent, the second had partially passed off by the hepatic ducts into the duodenum, and the third was intact; the greater part of the colon was sound, except at the point at which the liver was adherent, when it was covered with small ulcerations; the other viscera were sound; the right lung was compressed, from the increased size of the liver; the abscess apparently burst into the colon on the 25th. (*Annesley*, ibid, vol. i, *p.* 562.)

No. 150.—T. Donacliff, æt. 20, 4 months in India, admitted Oct. 29th, 1816, with pain in the abdomen, and purging; he had been ill for some days, and had been drinking freely. The subsequent symptoms were vomiting of dark-green bilious matter, with much soreness over the abdomen, but no particular pain; the stools were dysenteric, at times green, feculent, and scanty, and he also passed large portions of the mucous coat of the intestine; the skin was rather dry, with a greasy feel; the tongue dry, loaded, and red towards the apex; the pulse small and frequent. Leeches and blisters, together with salines and aperients, formed the main treatment. For the last week of his life there was constant, distressing, and obstinate hiccup, stupor, and a sense of weight in the head. Partial derangement preceded death, Nov. 13th.

Autopsy.—The liver was much enlarged, and studded throughout with small abscesses containing a very thick and semi-fluid pus, of a greenish-yellow colour; the substance of the liver was congested and inflamed; there was sloughy ulceration throughout the large intestines; and one ulcer in the colon had perforated the coats, allowing the contents of the intestine to escape into the abdominal cavity, where it had given rise to general peritonitis; the small intestines matted together and much displaced; the vessels of the mesentery amazingly turgid. (*Annesley*, ibid, vol. i, *p.* 563.)

No. 151.—H. Macklin, æt. 28, admitted April 25th, with chronic hepatitis. The remarkable feature in this case was the absence of most of those symptoms which are usually considered indicative of hepatic abscess; there were no tremors or rigors; pressure over the liver caused no pain, although there was evident fulness over the region of the liver; he could lie on either side with perfect ease; the bowels were for the most part, regular; he slept pretty well, and a few days before death, he walked up and down the ward; in addition to this, ptyalism was established; the symptoms which indicated the existence of abscess were tumefaction of the side, occasional cold sweats, great depression of spirits, hiccup, and indescribable languor. The tongue, at first foul, became subsequently much cleaner, and rather dry, with a white streak down each side; pulse from 80 to 120, full, soft, quick; urine high coloured at first; some vomiting of greenish bilious matter at the commencement, but this soon subsided.

Autopsy.—The right lobe of the liver adherent to the space between the 5th and 6th ribs, and formed a complete cyst, with a membranous lining, holding 90 ounces of watery and curdled matter; the small and large intestines perfectly sound; the pancreas was very much enlarged and hardened, and pressed upon the ductus communis choledicus and the other ducts, so as almost to prevent the passage of bile; the walls of the ducts were much thickened, and a cartilaginous band constricted this part. (*Annesley*, ibid, vol. i, *p.* 567.)

No. 152.—W. Harris, æt. 43, 25 years in India, admitted March 19th, 1817, with weakness of the knees from rheumatism, and vertigo. Mercurials were given early in the case, latterly nitrous acid and cinchona; the chief features of the case were pain in the right side under the cartilages of the ribs, affecting the respiration; "a severe stitch in the side;" a general sensation of heat; much flatulence and hiccup; tongue clean, smooth, chopped; pulse from 78 to 88, soft, irregular; latterly profuse sweats; urine very high coloured; stools very varied, sometimes red and watery, with a muddy sediment, at others watery, green, and mucous; there was no pain in the side on pressure; the abdomen became much distended with flatus, but without pain or uneasiness. He died April 3d.

Autopsy.—Liver enormous, occupying the whole of the epigastric and iliac regions; in the right lobe were five distinct abscesses; in the left lobe, on its concave surface, one abscess; this latter was adherent to the stomach, which was in a highly inflamed state. The five abscesses in the right lobe, contained nearly a pint of pus each, partly well formed, thick, and white, partly watery and coagulated, and part was of a yellowish-green hue, as if mixed with bile; colon and cæcum softened and ulcerated; small intestines of a dark, bluish colour; gall-bladder full of pale greenish-yellow bile, and as large as the urinary bladder when filled with urine; ducts pervious. (*Annesley*, ibid, vol. i, *p.* 571.)

No. 153.—Juntiman, long ill with dysentery and hepatitis, admitted from an out-station, and died the day after his arrival. History of the case not given.

Autopsy.—The right lobe of the liver rose up in a globular form in the right thorax, and contained an immense abscess filled with healthy pus; the substance of the liver was impacted, inflamed, and stretched across the abscess; the walls consisted entirely of the substance of the lobe, without any distinct cyst; they presented a smooth mucous tissue, insensibly passing into the condensed and impacted parenchymatous tissue. State of the intestines not given. (*Annesley*, ibid, vol. i, *p.* 567.)

No. 154.—Dr. J., ill many months with dysentery.. History of the case not given. Died Sept. 17th, 1821.

Autopsy.—Two abscesses in the liver, one on the superior convex part, adherent to the diaphragm, the other on the lateral portion, adhering to the ribs; the gall-bladder half full of dark bile, and the ducts compressed by knotty tumours and cellular adhesions; the stomach and duodenum congested; ilium softened, pulpy and contracted; colon of a dark colour externally, with ulcerations through the coats, by which the contents passed into the pelvis. (*Annesley*, vol. i, *p.* 577.)

No. 155.—Wood, long ill with chronic hepatitis and dysentery; died Jan. 5th, 1817. History not given.

Autopsy.—Liver enlarged, dark, hard, and gristly, and cut with difficulty, adherent to the diaphragm and ribs; the right lobe was one extensive abscess, the walls of which were white, hard, and perfectly cartilaginous; right lung adherent to the diaphragm, with some effusion in the right thorax; gall-bladder contained a little dark-green ropy bile; small intestines sound; the mucous coat of the large intestines inflamed. (*Annesley*, vol. i, *p.* 578.)

No. 156.—McMahon, admitted with dysentery, July 24th, 1816. Under the use of mercurials with other remedies, the dysentery subsided; but soon after, he had pain in the side, difficulty of breathing, and other symptoms of hepatitis. Bleeding, blisters, and mercury were used without effect. The disease terminated fatally.

Autopsy.—Liver very large, adherent to the diaphragm, contained two abscesses, one at the upper convex surface, nearly where the suspensory ligaments pass betwixt the right and left lobes, containing eight ounces of pus; the other was in the centre of the right lobe, and had "thick walls." Condition of the intestines not given. (*Annesley*, vol. i, *p.* 579.)

No. 157.—W. Schofield, æt. 29, admitted July 10th, with abdominal pain and vomiting, with much flatus, and a bitter taste in the mouth. The subsequent symptoms were principally, pain in the right side, distention of the abdomen, with an obscure tumour in the right hypochondrium; constant nausea and vomiting at first, inability to lie on the left side without a dragging sensation and pain, dysuria, lowness of spirits, with heaviness of looks, excessive thirst, and a rapid pulse; the tongue, at first white and dry, became gradually cleaner, and the character of the stools appears almost daily to have improved; from being highly bilious and morbid, they became "better" on August 7th, "infinitely more natural" on the 22d, and "perfectly natural" on the 26th. On the day before death, (August 31st,) he passed a perfectly natural motion, accompanied however by some coagula of blood. Treatment. Leeches, calomel in large doses, mercurial frictions, purgatives, &c.

Autopsy.—Liver very large, filling the whole of the epigastrium, and completely covering the stomach and colon, so as to prevent any part of them from being seen. It weighed six pounds, and was studded throughout with small abscesses containing thick matter; they had no cysts, and the tissue surrounding them was not more vascular and inflamed than any other part; some of these abscesses were very superficial, and elevated the external coat of the liver in the form of white tubercles; large intestines much contracted; colon filled with deep sloughing ulcers; large polypus in the right ventricle and auricle of the heart. (*Annesley*, vol. i, *p.* 502.)

No. 158.—W. Bates, long ill with hepatic derangement, and subsequently with a deranged state of the bowels and dysentery. History not given.

Autopsy.—Liver studded throughout with small abscesses, intermingled with light-brown coloured tubercles of a gristly nature, which, when divided, emitted a glairy fluid; colon filled with gangrenous ulcers, some of which had perforated the coats, and the escaped contents had given rise to much inflammation; small intestines and omentum matted together; the ilium, on its mucous coat, was ulcerated to the extent of four inches; gall-bladder empty; stomach and spleen healthy. (*Annesley*, vol. i, *p.* 511.)

No. 159.—Lieut. S., having been ill with fever, which had now subsided; admitted August 20th, 1820. The countenance was peculiar and sallow, the respiration impeded and oppressed; he could not lie with ease on either side; there was stinging sharp pain in the side, between the 5th and 6th right ribs, extending to the shoulder, and much augmented by pressure and deep inspiration; it was most severe at the posterior part of the liver near the spine; he had likewise pain in the right iliac region; the stools were watery, brown, and offensive; urine not high coloured; skin hot, with a greasy feel; pulse 120, hard; much thirst; no sleep. At no time had he rigors, vomiting, or cold sweats. Fluctuation becoming evident, the abscess was opened, but he died six hours afterwards, Sept. 13th. Mercury, externally and internally, failed to affect the system.

Autopsy.—Five large abscesses in the right lobe of the liver, viz. one which had been punctured; another adjoining, separated only by a thin septum; a third, in the posterior portion, adhering near the spine, and communicating by a very small opening with the opened abscess; the fourth was in the superior convex surface, adhering closly to the diaphragm, and the fifth was at the inferior margin of the right lobe, and adherent to the cæcum and head of the colon; the left lobe was sound, and all the other viscera seemed healthy. Case lxiv, in List of Operations. (*Annesley*, ibid, vol. i, *p.* 661.)

No. 160.—J. Gambell, æt. 23, admitted June 30th, with pain in the right side, very acute on pressure, considerable fulness at the epigastrium, with some cough; mercury was used externally and internally, with little benefit. The subsequent symptoms were cold sweats, a moist and sallow state of the skin, and urgent thirst; pulse 100, soft, full; tongue white and excited, latterly much cleaner; the respiration was hurried and impeded, the pain in the liver much increased by pressure, or by lying on the back; a tumour presented itself in the side, it was large and painful; this was opened, but with no benefit; he died five days afterwards, July 25th, in a state of delirium; the stools previous to the operation were very morbid, copious, and of a dark colour like clay, but afterwards they became perfectly white, and totally deficient of bile. At no period were there rigors or pain in the shoulder; early in the disease there was some dysuria, but the urine was natural.

Autopsy.—The whole of the left, and part of the right lobe formed a complete sac for the abscess; the gall-bladder completely adhered to the walls of the abscess, and communicated with it; the ducts were impervious, being involved in the adhesive inflammation of the parts forming the parietes of the abscess, and the bile secreted by the liver was either retained in the abscess or discharged by the wound, (this accounts for the characters of the stools.) The remaining portion of the liver was highly congested, and full of black blood; there was no disease in any of the other viscera. Case lxv, in List of Operations. (*Annesley,* ibid, *p.* 665.)

No. 161.—J. Day, admitted May 27th, 1817, with abdominal pain and dysentery; the symptoms of the latter were so severe as to mask, in a great measure, the existence of hepatic disease; he had no cold sweats, and there was no appearance of enlargement of the liver, nor was pain complained of, till near death, when much fulness was perceptible in this region; mercury was given freely, but nothing beyond a tender state of the gums was induced. He died June 2d.

Autopsy.—Liver much enlarged, with four abscesses in the right lobe, two on the convex surface, and a large one on the concave side; the latter had burst, and its contents escaped into the abdominal cavity; ulcerations in cæcum and rectum; small intestines thickened and white; heart enlarged, with white spots upon the right ventricle. (*Annesley*, ibid, vol. ii, *p*. 214.)

No. 162.—W. Carr, admitted Dec. 24th, with dysentery; on the 3d day after admission he had a slight fit of shivering, and this returned daily for several days; it was not followed by either heat or sweating; ptyalism was established; subsequently, there was much distention of the abdomen with hiccough, and pain in the course of the colon; (but he never complained of pain in the region of the liver;) vomiting of green viscid bilious matter, which was constant and distressing towards death, features sharpened, pulse rapid, tongue white in the centre, and latterly covered with dark mucus; the stools at various dates are reported "copious, tenacious, light,"—"green, mucous, fetid,"—"fetid and bloody,"—"scanty, like the sediment of coffee or chocolate." He died Jan. 15th.

Autopsy.—Liver enlarged, structure natural; on the convex surface of the right lobe was an encysted abscess containing 2 ounces of pus; gall-bladder full of yellow bile; small intestines healthy; colon adherent to the liver and spleen; its mucous coat and that of the rectum, corrugated and hanging in shreds; other viscera healthy. (*Annesley*, vol. ii, *p*. 217.)

No. 163.—G. Lush, æt. 29, admitted April 11th, 1819, with hepatitis, for which V. S., mercury, and purgatives were employed. On May 1st, the report is, "Mouth sore, no pain, but considerable enlargement under the right ribs; for 19 days after admission the bowels were rather bound; ptyalism was fully established, but no advantage was derived from it in reducing the size of the liver; dysenteric symptoms now appeared, and increased as the ptyalism decreased; this was after the man had been in hospital for three weeks. From the corrugated state of the membranous cyst enclosing the abscess, it was manifest that the abscess had been of a much larger size, and part of its contents removed by absorption after the supervention of the dysenteric symptoms; the subsidence of the tumefaction, which was evident in the right hypochondrium previous to the appearance of the dysenteric disorder, confirms this opinion." The chief symptoms were tumefaction of the side, which subsided as the disease advanced, a sense of weight or pain on lying on the left side, or on turning; vomiting, latterly; occasional pain in the liver, severe headache, hiccup, cold sweats, and much thirst; bowels very irregular; at no period was there cough or pain in the shoulder. He died May 25th.

Autopsy.—Liver rather large; one small abscess enclosed in a membranous cyst, in the centre of the right lobe; left lobe healthy, but pale; colon and cæcum ulcerated; rectum a mass of rugged ulceration; stomach and small intestines, pale and flaccid. (*Annesley*, ibid, vol. ii, *p.* 221.)

No. 164.—Bingham, admitted May 20th, with griping pain in the abdomen, pain in the right side, and sanguineous stools; these symptoms yielded several times to purgatives, mercurials, and blisters, but as often returned; hectic fever, and purging through the night, were present for several weeks before death. Appetite good to the last.

Autopsy.—One abscess in the superior part of the liver had penetrated through the diaphragm, and much purulent matter had escaped into the right lung, which was firmly adherent to the diaphragm; colon ulcerated throughout. (*Annesley*, ibid, vol. ii, *p.* 226.)

No. 165.—S. McDonald, of regular habits, admitted Sept. 1816, passing frequent muco-sanguineous stools, unattended by tenesmus or abdominal pain; he bore pressure without complaint, even over the liver; he had much vomiting, prostration of strength, and depression of spirits, with an increase of fever towards evening. Treatment not given.

Autopsy.—A large abscess on the concave surface of the right lobe of the liver; colon and cæcum ulcerated. (*Annesley*, ibid, vol. ii, *p.* 227.)

No. 166.—Martin, admitted April 22d, with dysenteric symptoms, which were so severe as to mask, in great measure, the hepatic affection; there was no pain in the liver, even on pressure, no pain in the shoulder, and only slight fulness in the hepatic region; stools very varied; latterly much vomiting of bilious matter, and he passed per anum large portions of the mucous coat of the intestine; skin natural, though he had cold sweats latterly; pulse 100 to 120, soft and full, tongue furred at the base, appetite quite gone; he became very weak; the body had a fetid smell, and for some hours before death, (May 22d,) he passed much black coagulated blood. Mercury entered largely into the treatment.

Autopsy.—Liver much enlarged, and studded throughout with small and distinct abscesses about the size of peas; the large intestines, from caput coli to rectum, one mass of ulceration. (*Annesley*, ibid, vol. ii, *p.* 227.)

No. 167.—J. Fagan, long ill with dysentery; he was apparently improving, when after exposure to the night air, he had a sudden shivering fit; from this date, (Oct. 6th) to that of his death

(Oct. 13th) he gradually became worse; he had no pain in the region of the liver, but he had severe pain in both shoulders, particularly in the right one; the stools were thin, yellow, and watery, passed without tenesmus or tormina; skin soft and moist, pulse 96 to 116, tongue moist but chopped; emaciation and debility advanced rapidly; no mention of the administration of mercury.

Autopsy.—The liver seemed sound and healthy, but on examination, a small abscess was discovered on the concave side of the left lobe; in the colon and rectum were some circumscribed ulcers, some of which had perforated the coats of the intestines; omentum much diseased and thickened; the other viscera sound. (*Annesley*, ibid, vol. ii, *p.* 361.)

No. 168.—R. Simpson, a Scotchman, æt. 38, 17 years in India, admitted with hepatitis, March 15th, died April 1st, 1838. Duration of disease 17 days. History of the case not given.

Autopsy.—In the concave side of the right lobe of the liver was a large abscess, whose walls, at one part, bore evidence of having long existed; whilst at others, they were rugged, and without any adventitious membrane whatever; the cellular tissue around was condensed and hard. (*Mr. Leith, Trans. of Med. and Phys. Soc. of Bombay*, vol. iv, *p.* 73.)

No. 169.—G. Jones, Englishman, æt. 36, 13¾ years in India, admitted with hepatitis, March 28th, died June 3d, 1839. History not given.

Autopsy.—An abscess in the left lobe of the liver; surrounding tissue degenerated. State of the intestines not given. (*Mr. Leith*, ibid, *p.* 73.)

No. 170.—E. Dunne, æt. 23, 4½ months in India, admitted with dysentery, for which he was bled, and took calomel till it affected his gums. Duration of the disease 60 days.

Autopsy.—Liver enlarged, with an abscess on its convex surface, and another at the lower margin of the left lobe; gall-bladder natural, colon contracted, with ulcerations on its mucous coat, cæcum, rectum, and small intestines healthy; mesenteric glands enlarged; right lung suppurating, adherent to the diaphragm; left lung healthy. (*Surg. Grant, Mad. Med. Journ.* vol ii, *p.* 213.)

No. 171.—G. Hethrington, æt. 23, 5 months in India, admitted with dysentery, for which he was bled freely and took calomel, but without effect. Duration of the disease 14 days.

Autopsy.—Liver, of natural size; right lobe dark slate colour, left lobe natural colour, tubercles dispersed throughout, and in the left lobe was also a small abscess containing several drachms of cheesy matter; patches of ulceration in colon, cæcum, and rectum; purulent effusion in the abdominal cavity; right lung adherent to the diaphragm and pleura. (*Surgeon Grant*, ibid.)

No. 172.—J. Blundell, sailor, æt. 25, admitted Dec. 10th, 1848, with hepatitis; he had great pain in the right side with extreme tenderness on pressure; he was bled, and took calomel till the mouth became very sore, but at this time a fulness became perceptible in the epigastrium, and soon afterwards he began to sweat profusely at nights; the bowels also became relaxed; fluctuation being evident, the abscess was opened, but he became very emaciated, and died Feb. 21st.

Autopsy.—Liver enlarged and pale; in the anterior surface of the right lobe, was an abscess; its cavity was nearly filled up, and the incision which had been made into it had united, and was marked by a cicatrix; mucous coat of colon in a state of sphacelas. Case lxxii in List of Operations. (*Dr. M. Stovell, Trans. of Med. and Phys. Soc. of Bombay*, No. 1, N. S. *p.* 163.)

No. 173.—Maria Duart, æt. 27, 9 years in India, three times in hospital during the previous six months, with hepatitis, for which she was salivated. On her last admission, June 6th, 1849, she had a small tumour in the right dorsal region, over the angles of the 7th and 8th ribs; this was opened, and there was a considerable discharge of pus evidently traceable to the liver. She gradually sank, and died Aug. 1st. No Autopsy. Case lxxiii in List of Operations. (*Dr. M. Stovell*, ibid, *p.* 164.)

No. 174.—G. Davis, sailor, æt. 26, 3 years in India, admitted Nov. 19th, 1849, with hepatitis; he had much pain, and some fulness in the right hypochondrium; he soon began to sweat profusely at nights; fluctuation becoming evident, the abscess was opened Dec. 1st; great temporary benefit ensued, but he became very exhausted, and died on the 14th Instant.

Autopsy.—Liver much enlarged, the right lobe nearly occupied by one large abscess, still containing much pus; the other abdominal and all the thoracic viscera normal. Case lxxiv in List of Operations. (*Dr. Stovell*, ibid, *p.* 164.)

No. 175.—T. Hewett, æt. 37, ill a month with hepatitis, admitted Dec. 19th, 1850. There was much fulness of the right side, and much emaciation; skin dry and hot; pulse 120, small and feeble; tongue moist, but coated down the centre; bowels irritable. The abscess was opened with temporary benefit, but he gradually sank, and died Jan. 3d. Treatment not given.

Autopsy.—Liver much enlarged; in the right lobe was the cavity of a large abscess, containing very little purulent matter; gall-bladder greatly distended; mucous coat of the large intestines dotted with small patches of ulceration; other viscera healthy. Case lxxv in List of Operations. (*Dr. Stovell*, ibid, *p.* 165.)

No. 176.—J. Carroll, sailor, æt. 20, 1 day in India, ill a month with hepatitis; there was tenderness and tumefaction in the right hypochondrium, countenance blanched and anxious, bowels irritable. Under the use of leeches, mercury, and opium he seemed to improve; the pain subsided, but not the tumefaction; the latter became more prominent, and fluctuation being felt, it was opened Sept. 3d. The discharge was free, but the bowels again became irritable; he had night sweats, loss of appetite, and much exhaustion. He died Sept. 27th. Mercury failed to affect the system.

Autopsy.—A large cavity in the right lobe of the liver, containing 8 ounces of thickish yellow pus; its walls uneven, rough, and indurated; colon thickened and ulcerated. Case lxxvi in List of Operations. (*Dr. Stovell*, ibid, *p.* 166.)

No. 177.—R. Farrow, æt. 39, often in hospital with hepatitis, admitted Oct. 27th, 1846. Previous to admission he was suddenly seized with vomiting, and also passed by a stool, a large quantity of pus, evidently from the bursting of an abscess into the intestines. He was very exhausted and died Nov. 8th. Treatment not given. No Autopsy. (*Dr. Stovell*, ibid, *p.* 166.)

No. 178.—Margaret Staunton, æt. 20, born in India, admitted July 10th, 1848, with hepatitis. She had great pain in the right hypochondrium, much increased on pressure, and a hot dry skin; she was bled, and took calomel till it affected the system, when the pain abated considerably. About a fortnight afterwards there was some fulness of the side, and she lost strength and flesh; the pain also returned, and she had sweats, with rapid exhaustion. On Aug. 25th, she passed much pus by stool, and this continued till near her death on Sept. 3d. No Autopsy. (*Dr. Stovell*, ibid, *p.* 167.)

No. 179.—L. Templan, æt. 30, 1 year in India, admitted Jan. 25th, 1849, with hepatitis, for which he was bled, and took opium, mercury, &c. He rapidly lost flesh and strength, and became so exhausted that on Feb. 2d, he was partially collapsed, though perfectly sensible. On the 4th, his abdomen became tympanitic, but he had no pain. He rapidly sank, and died on the 5th.

Autopsy.—A large abscess in the right lobe of the liver had burst, and discharged its contents into the abdominal cavity; the other viscera normal. The abscess apparently burst on the 2d Instant. (*Dr. Stovell*, ibid, *p.* 167.)

No. 180.—Amelia Scarles, æt. 34, born in India, admitted Oct. 6th, 1848, with hepatitis. She had much pain in the right side, increased on pressure; bowels irritable; pulse 108, small and depressed. Under the use of leeches, calomel, opium, &c., her health improved, although her mouth was not affected by mercury. On Nov. 3d, she was seized with cough and a sense of suffocation, and she expectorated much pus; this was followed by great depression, and she died on the 6th Instant.

Autopsy.—Liver enlarged, firm, granular; in the right lobe was an extensive abscess, which by a large opening, was discharging its contents into the bronchi; it still contained much thick pus; lower portion of the right lung slightly hepatized; intestines and other viscera healthy. (*Dr. Stovell*, ibid, *p.* 169.)

No. 181.—J. Burrows, æt. 24, 1 year in India, admitted Feb. 15th, 1849, with hepatitis. There was much pain in the hepatic region, and a hot dry skin. Under the use of leeches, &c., and mercury carried to the extent of distinctly affecting the mouth, the pain subsided, but some fulness remained. On March 2d, purulent expectoration commenced, his breathing became hurried, skin hot, tongue brown and dry, and pulse rapid and feeble. Delirium preceded his death on the 5th.

Autopsy.—A large abscess occupied nearly the whole lobe of the liver, a small portion only of the contents, having escaped into the bronchi; no other morbid appearances were observed. (*Dr. Stovell*, ibid, *p.* 170.)

No. 182.—Ann Keys, æt. 35, 8 years in India, admitted Sept. 19th, 1849, with hepatitis, for which she was bled, and took calomel till distinct ptyalism was established. She became much better, and went home Oct. 9th, but her stomach remained irritable. On the 23d, she was re-admitted, with a return of the pain. On the 26th of Nov., after a little coughing for the previous day or two, she expectorated much pus, and this continued till she died exhausted, Dec. 26th. No Autopsy. (*Stovell*, ibid.)

No. 183.—H. Nelson, bricklayer, æt. 26, 1 year in India, admitted Jan. 17th, 1852, with hepatitis, of which he had been ill from Dec. 20th. He had been freely leeched, and his system affected by mercury. On admission he was much reduced in strength, and there was dulness on percussion as high as the nipple, but he was quite free from pain; pulse 86, soft, and small; no improvement took place, and he had febrile accessions towards evening, terminating in profuse sweats. On Feb. 17th, he was suddenly seized with severe cough, and expectorated about 4 ounces of pus tinged with blood; this continued till his death, May 5th. Latterly his feet became œdematous, and his strength exhausted.

Autopsy.—The base of the lower lobe of the right lung adherent to the diaphragm; there was also adhesion between the diaphragm and the upper surface of the right lobe of the liver; the latter contained a large abscess, which had been discharging its contents into the bronchi, through an opening in the diaphragm; the left lobe and other viscera healthy, as was also the left lung. (*Dr. Stovell,* ibid, *p.* 176.)

No. 184.—M. Smith, Irishman, æt. 23, 1 year in India, admitted with a second attack of liver disease, and died in Aug. 1828, after 8 days stay in hospital. He had pain in the right side and shoulder, vomiting, fever, with a weak frequent pulse, a tendency to clammy sweats, and rapid sinking; the evacuations were unhealthy. The treatment in this and the 27 following cases not given.

Autopsy.—One large abscess in the right lobe of the liver near the diaphragm; the intestines vascular externally. (*Dr. Geddes, (Case 3) in Trans. of the Med. and Phys. Society of Calcutta,* vol. vi, *p.* 337, *and Clin. Illustrations of the Diseases of India, p.* 309.)

No. 185.—J. Sullivan, Irishman, æt. 21, 1 year in India, admitted with dysentery in July, and died in Aug. 1828, after ten days stay in hospital. This was a case of severe dysentery, with irregular exacerbations of hectic fever, and great debility; there was no pain in the side, nor in the shoulder, and only vomiting latterly; stools dysenteric.

Autopsy.—Numerous suppurating tubercles in the liver, together with much ulceration and thickening of the large intestines. (*Dr. Geddes.*)

No. 186.—H. McGuire, Irishman, æt. 21, 1 year in India, admitted with continued fever, and died after 40 days illness, in Sept. 1828. He had occasional vomiting, diarrhœa with unhealthy stools, pain in the side for 9 days preceding death, but no pain in the shoulder; hectic fever, and increasing debility.

Autopsy.—Abscess in the liver, large, solitary, deep-seated; the intestines healthy. (*Dr. Geddes.*)

No. 187.—P. McCarthy, Irishman, æt. 26, 2 years in India, 6 times previously treated for hepatitis; admitted with dysentery and liver disease, and died in September, after 11 days illness. There was pain in the right lumbar region, much constitutional disorder, with weak pulse, moist skin, and increasing debility; stools latterly dysenteric; no pain in the shoulder; no vomiting.

Autopsy.—One abscess, not large, on the margin of the right lobe of the liver, with adhesions to the colon; large intestines ulcerated from cæcum to rectum. (*Dr. Geddes.*)

No. 188.—J. Horme, Englishman, æt. 32, 7 years in India, admitted with debility and hectic fever in Sept., and died in Oct. 1828, having been ill 24 days. The most prominent feature was dysentery with increasing debility; no pain in the side or shoulder; no vomiting.

Autopsy.—Numerous small abscesses in the liver; the colon and cæcum ulcerated and thickened. (*Dr. Geddes.*)

No. 189.—P. Crowley, Irishman, æt. 35, 12 years in India, admitted with hepatitis and intermittent fever; died in January 1829, having been ill 20 days; it was his 13th admission with hepatic disease. He had pain in the right side and epigastrium, with accessions of fever, and great perspirations; also occasional vomiting, and pain in the shoulder on coughing; stools unhealthy, latterly with a little blood; there was jaundice on the 4th day previous to death.

Autopsy.—One large abscess in the centre of the right lobe, and a small one in the left; caput coli beginning to ulcerate. (*Dr. Geddes.*)

No. 190.—T. Galvin, Irishman, æt. 22, 2 years in India, admitted with a third attack of hepatitis, and died, after being ill 8 days, in March, 1829. At first he had pain at the scrobiculus cordis, but this soon left him; pain in the right shoulder, frequent vomiting, and profuse sweats; there was no affection of the intestines.

Autopsy.—One small abscess near the posterior part of the liver; the intestine healthy. (*Dr. Geddes.*)

No. 191.—T. Craddock, Englishman, æt. 28, 2⅓ years in India, admitted with his ninth attack of hepatic disease, and died in June, 1829, after 19 days illness. He had occasional pain near the right false ribs, pain in the shoulder, synochal fever at first, afterwards hectic, also sleeplessness, and much debility; no vomiting; no affection of the bowels.

Autopsy.—One large abscess in the upper and outer part of the right lobe of the liver; colon slightly contracted. (*Dr. Geddes.*)

No. 192.—J. Lyons, Englishman, æt. 28, 2½ years in India, admitted with the fifth attack of hepatic disease; he died in June, 1828, after being in hospital 15 days. He had pain in the site of the abscess and in the shoulder, hectic fever with evening exacerbations, and a small weak pulse, and frequent vomiting; bowels inclined to constipation; a somewhat sudden sinking preceded death.

Autopsy.—One large abscess in the upper part of the right lobe of the liver; colon contracted. (*Dr. Geddes.*)

No. 193.—P. Brophy, Irishman, æt. 27, 1 year in India, admitted with continued fever; died July, 1829, after being in hospital 44 days. He had fever, with oppression and vague pains about the chest; then, for a long time only a great feeling of weakness, want of appetite, and occasional evening exacerbations of fever; and subsequently, pain in the right lumbar region, with affection of the bowels, and latterly he passed a little blood; at no period was there pain in the shoulder, or vomiting.

Autopsy.—One large abscess in the inferior margin of the right lobe of the liver; intestines healthy. (*Dr. Geddes.*)

No. 194.—B. Asquoth, Englishman, æt. 22, 2 years in India, admitted with a fourth attack of diarrhœa; died July, 1829, after 37 days illness. He had at first diarrhœa with some pyrexia, afterwards occasional pain in the liver, and febrile exacerbations, eventually with great sweating; and a swelling was observed at the scrobiculus cordis, suddenly becoming more diffused, with aggravation of all the symptoms; no pain in the shoulder; vomiting frequent, especially latterly; bowels loose at first, afterwards irregular.

Autopsy.—In the left lobe of the liver was one large abscess, which had burst towards the concave surface, and its contents had escaped into the abdominal cavity. *A needle was found imbedded firmly in the centre of the right lobe, at a distance from the abscess.* In the colon were one or two round ulcers. (*Dr. Geddes.*)

No. 195.—T. Smith, Englishman, æt. 25, 2 years in India, admitted with hepatic disease in April, and died in August 1829, having been ill 118 days. He had occasional pain in the side and shoulder, generally no vomiting, hectic fever, perspirations, and gradual sinking; stools either dysenteric or of a pale yellow colour.

Autopsy.—One large abscess in the upper and outer part of the right lobe; contraction of portions of the colon. (*Dr. Geddes.*)

No. 196.—W. Clarke, Englishman, æt. 23, 3 years in India, admitted for the seventh time with hepatitis; died in Nov. 1829, after 90 days illness. He had pain in the side, severe pain in the shoulder at first, but afterwards none, hectic fever with febrile accessions, eventually discharge of matter by cough, and general sinking; stools loose, unhealthy, with, at times, streaks of blood; no vomiting.

Autopsy.—One large abscess in the upper part of the right lobe of the liver, communicating with the lungs; intestines healthy. (*Dr. Geddes.*)

No. 197.—J. Hoolahan, Irishman, æt. 20, 6 months in India, admitted with dysentery, and died after 80 days illness in Dec. 1829. Symptoms. Occasional pain in the side and shoulder, hectic fever, frequent rigors, gradual emaciation, debility, slight vomiting, and dysenteric stools.

Autopsy.—One large abscess in the upper part of the right lobe of the liver; large intestines ulcerated throughout. (*Dr. Geddes.*)

No. 198.—L. Farren, Irishman, æt. 21, 1¼ year in India, admitted with abdominal inflammation in Oct., and died in Dec., having been ill 70 days. He had pain below the scrobiculus cordis, with intervals of ease and general amendment of symptoms; these comprised hectic fever, a dysenteric state of the bowels, and occasional vomiting; eventually there was a diffused swelling over the stomach; no pain in the shoulder.

Autopsy.—Numerous small abscesses in the left lobe of the liver, and one large one extending to the middle lobe; large intestines ulcerated throughout. (*Dr. Geddes.*)

No. 199.—J. Bradshaw, Englishman, æt. 27, 6 months in India, admitted with pain in the side and dysentery; died in Jan. 1829, after 12 days illness. He had occasional pain in the side, with slight fever, loss of appetite, nausea, and occasional vomiting; then severe dysentery, with hectic fever; no pain in the shoulder.

Autopsy.—A few abscesses in both lobes of the liver, particularly in the upper part of the right lobe; large intestines ulcerated throughout. (*Dr. Geddes.*)

No. 200.—P. Moore, Irishman, æt. 31, 4 years in India, admitted with dysentery in Aug., and died in Oct., 1829, having been ill 56 days. He had at first, dysentery; then occasional pain in the side, and right lumbar region, with hectic, sweatings, vomiting, gradual emaciation, and œdema; no pain in the shoulder; stools dysenteric.

Autopsy.—One large abscess in the upper and outer side of the right lobe of the liver, and bounded by the diaphragm; intestines slightly diseased. (*Dr. Geddes.*)

No. 201.—G. Lee, Englishman, æt. 27, 4 years in India, admitted with an eighth attack of hepatic disease, and died in Nov. 1830, after 88 days illness. He had severe pain in the site of a swelling in the right hypochondrium, and also in the right shoulder; vomiting at the outset and towards the close of the case; irregular bowels, stools sometimes costive, at others loose, with blood; the abscess was opened, and matter evacuated: hectic with emaciation, and finally, convulsions preceded death.

Autopsy.—One large abscess in the outer part of the right lobe of the liver, penetrating between the ribs to the skin; intestines healthy. (*Dr. Geddes.*) No. 201 in List of Operations.

No. 202.—J. Quinlan, Irishman, æt. 25, 4 years in India, admitted with a second attack of hepatitis, and died in Jan. 1831, after 12 days illness. He had rigors, severe pain in the right lumbar region, at first diarrhœa, latterly dysentery, occasional vomiting, pyrexia, deafness, and much debility; no pain in the shoulder.

Autopsy.—One large abscess in the inferior margin of the right lobe of the liver, adherent to the colon; in this viscus, at the point of adhesion, were one or two superficial ulcers. (*Dr. Geddes.*)

No. 203.—J. Forster, æt. 23, 2 years in India, admitted with a ninth attack of hepatic disease, and died in April 1831, after 27 days illness. He had severe pain at first in the breast and other parts of the right side and also in the shoulder; rigors, cold sweats, hectic, and occasional vomiting; much dysentery, particularly towards death.

Autopsy.—One large abscess in the upper and posterior part of the right lobe of the liver; caput coli and rectum ulcerated. (*Dr. Geddes.*)

No. 204.—G. Bowman, Englishman, æt. 24, 4½ years in India, admitted with a second attack of hepatitis, and died in May 1831, after 13 days illness. Symptoms. Pain in the right side, occasional vomiting, dysentery latterly, much thirst, furred tongue, cool damp skin, and exhaustion; no pain in the shoulder.

Autopsy.—Numerous small abscesses, particularly in the right lobe, and a large one between the two lobes; there were ulcers in the cæcum, caput coli, and rectum. (*Dr. Geddes.*)

No. 205.—J. Hughes, Englishman, æt. 25, 5 years in India, admitted with hepatitis, and died in June 1831, after 11 days illness. Symptoms. Pain in the right lobe of the liver, anxiety, great perspiration, thirst, vague pains about the limbs, restlessness, oppression at the epigastrium, with frequent vomiting, and slight irregularity of the bowels; no pain in the shoulder.

Autopsy.—One large abscess in the upper and posterior part of the right lobe of the liver; intestines healthy. (*Dr. Geddes.*)

No. 206.—J. Bradshaw, Irishman, æt. 26, 4 years in India, admitted with dysentery, and died in Oct. 1831, after 43 days illness. There was no pain generally, only alluded to twice, long continued affection of the bowels, stools loose and dysenteric; occasional vomiting; slight yellowness of the eyes, irregular hectic sweats, gradual emaciation, and debility preceded death; no pain in the shoulder.

Autopsy.—One large abscess in the upper part of the right lobe of the liver, half an inch from the surface; superficial ulcers in the colon. (*Dr. Geddes.*)

No. 207.—T. Murphy, Irishman, æt. 33, 5 years in India, admitted with pain in the right lumbar region, and abdominal inflammation; died in Nov. 1831, after 63 days illness. He had steady pain below the epigastrium, much weakness and sweatings, with a quick small pulse; bowels loose, stools laterly sanguineous; no pain in the shoulder; no vomiting. There was an attack like cholera, and very gradual exhaustion, till death.

Autopsy.—One large abscess in the upper part of the right lobe of the liver; some ulceration with thickening, in the colon and rectum. (*Dr. Geddes.*)

No. 208.—J. Higham, Englishman, æt. 27, 2½ years in India, admitted with a sixth attack of hepatic disease; died Jan. 28th, after 28 days illness. He had pain in the liver and in the shoulder, very severe at times—frequent vomiting—hectic fever—and gradual emaciation with debility—stools loose, with blood and mucus sometimes.

Autopsy.—One large abscess in the upper and outer part of the right lobe of the liver; colon contracted, its mucous coat red and corrugated; no ulceration. (*Dr. Geddes.*)

No. 209.—T. Hurst, Englishman, æt. 27, 2½ years in India, admitted with a third attack of hepatic disease; died Jan. 1832, after 10 days stay in hospital. For two months he had occasional pain in the hepatic region, with rigors, perspirations, frequency of pulse, loss of appetite, sleeplessness, and gradual emaciation; then severe dysenteric symptoms; and, for ten days before death, expectoration of purulent matter. At first there was pain in the cardiac region, and also occasionally in the right shoulder; no vomiting.

Autopsy.—One abscess at the posterior and upper part of the right lobe of the liver, penetrating the right crus of the diaphragm, and the lungs; numerous transverse ulcers in the colon. (*Dr. Geddes.*)

No. 210.—An Englishman, æt. 24, 3¾ years in India, admitted with hepatitis, and died in May, 1832, after 23 days illness. At first there were stitches in the right hypochondrium, and then a swelling appeared at the edge of the ribs, which increased with gradual exhaustion, emaciation, and weakness, but little pain; there was also vomiting and pain in the shoulder; stools latterly loose and unhealthy.

Autopsy.—One large abscess in the right lobe of the liver, extending below the ligamentum latum into the left lobe; intestines healthy. (*Dr. Geddes, p.* 319.)

No. 211.—An Irishman, æt. 27, $5\frac{3}{4}$ years in India, admitted with hepatitis; died in Oct. 1832, after 16 days treatment. He had severe pain in the right side and shoulder, gradually lessening till the sixth day; then frequent vomiting, sweats, weakness, and exhaustion; eyes tinged yellow, pulse contracted, urine high coloured, stools vitiated.

Autopsy.—One large abscess in the upper and outer part of the right lobe of the liver; intestines healthy. (*Dr. Geddes.*)

No. 212.— ——, admitted with hepatic disease, and died in July, 1830, after a stay in hospital of 192 days. It commenced with pain in the right side and shoulder, gradually passing more into the right breast; latterly cough, and expectoration streaked with blood, inability to lie except on the left side, hectic, emaciation, vomiting; bowels at first loose, then more regular.

Autopsy.—One large abscess on the upper surface of the right lobe of the liver; intestines healthy. (*Dr. Geddes.*)

No. 213— ——, æt. 39, 10 years in India, recently ill with "spasm of the bowels," admitted May 18th, 1820, with severe and heavy pain in the right side, increased by motion, pressure, and full inspiration; pulse 89, not hard; skin warm and moist; tongue sizy, white. Under the use of leeches, calomel, &c., he seemed to improve, but the stools became like coffee on June 18th, and he died next day.

Autopsy.—A large abscess in the centre of the liver containing 24 ounces of thin coffee-like fluid with flakes of pus; another small abscess on the right lobe held 2 ounces of healthy pus; some patches of engorgement in large intestines; no other morbid appearance. (*Dr. Conwell on the Liver, p.* 490.)

No. 214.—A Sepoy, æt. 25, long ill with dysentery, and subsequently with an herpetic eruption, and pains in the extremities, admitted July 5th, 1825. Symptoms. Cutaneous eruptions, general debility, emaciation, loss of appetite, little sleep from pains and purging, stools yellow or dark, face bloated, distention of abdomen after eating; thorax deformed by increased convexity, with dyspnæa, and dulness on percussion. He died Sept. 3d. Treatment chiefly palliative, with an alterative course of mercury.

Autopsy.—Liver dense (carneous) and dark; in the right lobe an abscess containing 26 ounces of fluid resembling chocolate, and 4 ounces of curdiform matter; the sac lined by a fleecy membrane resembling chamois leather, one-sixth of an inch thick, and in parts cartilaginous; bile flowed freely into the sac without any pressure; gall-bladder large and full, adherent to the colon, and contained bile and pus; no ulceration of the large intestines; mucous coat of small intestines thickened; mesenteric glands enlarged and pale; softening of the brain and spine. (*Dr. Conwell,* ibid, *p.* 491.)

No. 215.— ——, æt. 40, 25 years in India, robust, healthy, ill for the first time in India, admitted Oct. 27th, 1826, with purging. The symptoms were very obscure till just before death; he only complained of pain from hæmorrhoids; abdominal pressure gave no uneasiness, but there was a great sense of fulness and heaviness about the rectum and neck of the bladder; he had craving appetite, and a constant sense of emptiness; his spirits were good, and he laughed, a little before his death, at the idea of being in danger; he occasionally passed worms, (tænia and ascarides,) also portions of the intestine, and latterly a large coagulum of blood; the day before death, the stools were coffee-coloured; latterly he had cold sweats, much thirst, and cold extremities; tongue red, pulse 100 to 140; countenance anxious. He died suddenly, Nov. 20th. Treatment. Leeches, calomel, opium, ipecacuanha, the warm bath, &c.

Autopsy.—Liver much enlarged, dense and fatty; contained in various parts eighteen abscesses; four large, the other the size of hazel nuts; omentum adherent to the liver, aiding to cover an abscess, which contained thin coffee-coloured fluid with yellow curdiform flakes; large intestines ulcerated throughout; likewise the whole length of the ilium; in the latter were two tænia, 7 feet long; perforations in the cæcum and colon; mucous coat of the stomach dark and corrugated, that of the duodenum and jejunum with patches of engorgement; spleen pale and small; kidneys natural; mesentery very fat; pancreas small, dark, and congested. (*Dr. Conwell,* ibid, *p.* 493.)

No. 216.— ——, æt. 39, 3 years in India, fair, tall, thin, healthy, admitted July 17th, 1828, with pain in the abdomen increased on pressure; purging with tenesmus, heaviness, and fulness; skin warm and clammy, pulse 100, tongue dry and brown. No further history given; died July 25.

Autopsy.—Liver much enlarged, pale, very granular, two small abscesses in the right lobe, the larger in the centre of the lobe held 4 ounces of dark pus; the surface of the cyst presented a series of white and yellow flocculi, the remains of organized vessels and nerves (?)—gall-bladder contained half an ounce of very viscid granular bile. *The kidneys had some vascular congestion, and pus was observed issuing from the mammillary processes of the left one.* Spleen small and flaccid; ilium ulcerated, especially near its cæcal extremity; colon and cæcum much ulcerated, some ulcers sloughing, others in an early stage of ulceration. (*Dr. Conwell*, ibid, *p.* 496.)

No. 217.——, æt. 22, 8 months in India, middle stature, muscular, fair, ruddy, of irregular habits, admitted April 16th, 1827, having been discharged only 17 days before, when he had been treated for purging and abdominal pains. On admission, he was much emaciated and weak, eyes sunk, countenance collapsed; pain in the chest and epigastrium, also in the shoulders and extremities; nausea; loss of appetite; much thirst; stools frequent, yellow, watery; urine dark and scanty; fauces dry, slightly impeding speech; pulse 120, soft and small; tongue furred with irregular transverse sulci, and enlarged red papillæ; skin moist and cool. Subsequently the hepatic enlargement increased, the breathing became hurried, the tongue became quite clean, of a scarlet-red colour, yet preserving the angular sulci, and at last it became dry and ulcerated; urine dark till near death, when it became pale, but blended with a thick white deposit that rendered it opaque when agitated. Mercury in large doses failed to produce ptyalism. Hectic with night sweats, sleeplessness, and pains in the trunk, shoulders, and extremities preceded death, May 19th.

Autopsy.—Liver much enlarged; in it three abscesses, one near its superior, and two near its inferior surface, containing 16 oz. of pus; gall-bladder contained some thin orange-coloured bile; kidneys dark, congested; pancreas dark; patches of engorgement in the ilium; large intestines extensively ulcerated, in parts sphacelated; lungs congested; serous effusion in the skull and spinal cord; heart healthy. (*Dr. Conwell*, ibid, *p.* 297.)

No. 218.—A Sailor, æt. 26, of irregular habits, subject to syphilis, for which he had taken mercury freely, admitted July 27th, with purging. The subsequent symptoms were pain in the "back," loss of appetite, much thirst, sleeplessness; urine copious like decoction of cinchona, muco-sanguineous or bilio-feculent; pulse rapid, tongue furred, no abdominal pain throughout, but soreness; cold perspirations, stools like coffee grounds; confused ideas, restlessness, and startings in the sleep preceded his death, August 9th.

Autopsy.—Liver congested, with numerous points containing pus in small cysts, from the size of a millet seed to that of a pea, throughout both the right and left lobes; liver adherent to the colon; on separating this, a large abscess was found in the right lobe; *pressure of the kidneys showed pus passing from the tubuli uriniferi into the infundibulum on each side;* mucous coat of stomach flaccid, with points of ecchymosis; in the ilium numerous ulcers; these were more numerous and extensive near the cæcum; deep ulceration throughout the colon and rectum; in the head was some sub-arachnoid effusion; lungs congested; the lining of the aorta, slight pink throughout. (*Dr. Conwell*, ibid, *p.* 500.)

No. 219.— ——, æt. 45, slender, emaciated, ill 40 days with fever, constant dry cough, and pains in the right side and shoulder; admitted July 7th, 1827. The acute symptoms were then abated, but there was great debility, and frequent purging; skin cold and clammy, urine scanty red or dark, pulse 120, thready and soft, loss of appetite, sleeplessness, and fulness and soreness in the hepatic region. Died July 8th. Treatment palliative.

Autopsy.—Liver enlarged; its tissue dense, close, carneous, adherent to the diaphragm; at this point was an abscess containing 11 ounces of nearly colourless fluid and flaky pus. There was a second abscess on the posterior surface of the right lobe, and two others on the convex and superior surface; the abscess-walls were of a yellowish colour, and of uneven surface, and on filling them with water, numerous flocculi floated in it; some of these flocculi were easily detached, others adhered firmly to their bases; gall-bladder contained 2 ounces of greenish-yellow viscid bile; spleen small and pale; pancreas large and dark; 17 living lumbrici in the ilium; mucous coat of the stomach rather pale; that of the duodenum of a slate colour; that of the ilium congested and ulcerated; the ilio-cæcal valve destroyed by ulceration; the whole of the large intestines a mass of ulceration, in parts sphacelated; right lung adherent to the side, left one natural. (*Dr. Conwell*, ibid, *p.* 503.)

No. 220.— ——, æt. 22, long ill with dysentery, for which he had been salivated; admitted July 14th, died on the 29th instant, 1827. Symptoms. Great debility, emaciation, fulness and pain in the epigastrium, nausea, vomiting, and jaundice with copious clay-coloured stools; pulse 108, small, feeble; tongue furred; skin cool and clammy; urine like stale decoction of cinchona, and opaque. He stated that his earliest symptoms were pains in the back, afterwards sickness of the stomach, and then dysentery. Cold sweats, low delirium, and coma preceded his death.

Autopsy.—Liver enlarged; in its centre a large abscess containing 8 pints of aqueous coffee-coloured fluid, blended with pus; it had entirely removed the lobulus spigelii, and formed its own parietes by false membranes and adhesions to the stomach. There were several other small cysts containing dark fluid and pus; in the gall-bladder was ½ ounce of thin green bile; *pressure forced pus from the mammillary processes of the kidneys;* the mucous coat of the stomach, opposite the adhesion to the liver, was ulcerated; small intestines congested; cæcal extremity of the ilium ulcerated; transverse arch of the colon and rectum ulcerated; in the right lung were numerous minute tubercles filled with pus; the lining of the ascending aorta of a deep yellow colour; congestion of the brain with much serous effusion. (*Dr. Conwell*, ibid, *p.* 505.)

No. 221.— ——, æt. 22, taken ill with pain in the head and fever, Oct. 19th; he was bled, and he took mercurials till the 25th, when he complained of hepatic pain, and passed frequent mucous stools. Subsequently there was much emaciation, abdominal and epigastric pain on pressure, anorexia, and sleeplessness; there was no pain in the liver latterly; stools frequent, muco-sanguineous, occasionally with coagula of blood; urine scanty; pulse 98, quick, and small; skin warm, with much perspiration. Died Nov. 19th.

Autopsy.—Liver dark, with abscess in the right lobe, which contained 16 ounces of pus; left lobe seemed gritty when incised. Large intestines congested and ulcerated throughout, in parts sphacelated; lungs congested, heart pale and flaccid, with serous effusion (5½ oz.) in the pericardium. (*Dr. Conwell,* ibid, *p.* 507.)

No. 222.— ——, admitted with dysentery, passing blood and mucus; pulse 120, small and hard; skin cold and moist; tongue marked by sulci. Exhaustion, sinking, and coma preceded death, June 16th. Treatment. Blue-pill, ipecacuanha, opium, &c.

Autopsy.—Liver contained four extensive abscesses, a large branch of the hepatic vein traversed the largest superiorly, and part of its coats were removed by ulceration; pus and mucus occupied the calibre of this part, and a coagulum of blood filled the cavity of the tube nearest to the biliary acini; the contents of the abscesses were dark, and some bile mingled with each. "Sundry corrugations, covered with thick layers or false membrane, indicate the probable site of previous hepatic abscesses"(?) Mucous coat of small intestines pale, except the ilium, which was congested; thence to the rectum a mass of ulceration; kidneys small and pale; spleen and pancreas dark. (*Dr. Conwell,* ibid, *p.* 508.)

No. 223.— ——, æt. 26, 3 years in India, twice in two months ill with dysentery; admitted Dec. 30th. He had suffered for five days from a succession of chills and flushes; he had also pain and heaviness about the stomach, thirst, anorexia, and sleeplessness; pulse 78, small and feeble; skin hot; tongue furred; he passed pus in his urine occasionally, at intervals of several days; purging set in, and he died in Feb. Treatment. Calomel, ipecacuanha, blisters, leeches, &c.

Autopsy.—Liver enlarged, weighing 8 pounds, adherent to the diaphragm; in the right lobe a large abscess, containing 2½ pounds of matter, one-half of which was a dark, watery fluid, and the other half dark, flaky, curdiform pus; the walls were uneven, and when scraped, were observed to be pierced with foramina of different sizes; a small probe was passed into one, which was found to be the opening of a branch of the hepatic vein leading to the vena cava; gall-bladder thickened, diminished, and contained bile and pus; the spleen, pancreas and kidneys all diminished in size; the mucous coat of the small intestines congested; the lower extremity of the ilium, and also the cæcum, colon, and rectum presented large transverse ulcerated fissures. (*Dr. Conwell*, ibid, *p*. 510.)

No. 224.— ——, æt. 30, 7 years in India, tall, muscular, extremely intemperate; admitted Aug. 15th, 1831, with pain across the abdomen, and purging; stools frequent, mucous, and passed with tenesmus. Pains in the right shoulder, the limbs, and the diaphragm were complained of, but he stated that these were of two years duration, and for them he had taken mercurials and other remedies. These pains were first regarded as rheumatic, but subsequently the pulse became compressed and quick; this, with other circumstances, altered the diagnosis; tongue sulcated in all directions. On Oct. 9th and 10th he passed purulent urine; this afterwards changed to a red colour; copious muco-purulent expectoration, dyspnæa, and much pain in the side preceded death, Nov. 30th.

Autopsy.—Liver small and pale, with an irregular surface like a citron; an abscess in the superior and posterior part of the right lobe, its sac consisting of organized lymph ¾ of an inch thick; it had burst through the diaphragm into the right thorax, which was filled with light coffee-coloured fluid with flakes of pus; the lung was perfectly hepatized or carneous, and it lay flat to the spine, reduced to the size of a middle-sized muscle; in the ilium were patches of congestion and ulceration; the mucous coat of the large intestines was prodigiously thickened, smooth, and red, resembling muscular tissue throughout; spleen small and pale, kidneys natural size but congested, some small ulcerations in the bladder near the openings of the ureters. (*Dr. Conwell*, ibid, *p*. 512.)

No. 225.— ——, æt. 46, 25 years in India, very subject to hepatitis and dysentery from habitual excesses; died Sept. 8th, 1831. Symptoms. Pain across the abdomen increased on pressure; purging, stools frequent, muco-sanguineous, passed with tormina and tenesmus; pulse 88, soft, tongue furred white, skin cool and moist, urine free. From the commencement he seemed quite overcome, moaned heavily, complained of extreme debility; before death he passed several coagula of blood in his stools; mercury was given largely and unremittingly, but it failed to affect the system, although it made the gums sore.

Autopsy.—Liver dark-coloured, congested, contained two abscesses, one in the inferior and posterior surface, the other in the centre; both contained thick pus; there was an irregular cicatrix on the right convex surface. Ulcers in various stages in cæcum, colon, and rectum; slight pulmonary engorgement. (*Dr. Conwell*, ibid, *p.* 515.)

No. 226.— ——, æt. 24, 11 months in India, middle size, sickly; ill two months, with a frequent, dry cough; admitted Sept. 24th, 1831. Pulse 92, soft; skin cool, tongue clean, bowels regular, urine natural; great thirst, no appetite; the cough and febrile symptoms became gradually aggravated, expectoration copious, streaked with blood; complaint supposed to be pulmonary, and treated as such; emaciation, occasional febrile attacks, and copious sweats preceded his death, which took place suddenly, Dec. 7th. Treatment. Leeches, setons, mercurials, aperients, &c.

Autopsy.—Lungs congested; in the inferior lobe of the right lung was a small abscess, into which the bronchi opened; it had no apparent communication with the hepatic abscess. Liver large, weighing 5 pounds, adherent to the diaphragm, which formed superiorly, the parietes of an abscess in the liver, holding 19 ounces of pus; the abscess contained a large coagulum of blood, surrounded by pus, and numerous little bloody clots adherent to the projecting points of the surface; these projections were the extremities of eroded arteries, and the tubular form was traced in some, the extremities being closed by a clot of red blood; the abscess was crossed or traversed by shreds or flocculi, apparently the debris of vessels; these floated on all sides when the sac was filled with water; the hepatic tissue mottled white and dark. Condition of the intestines not stated. "The hæmorrhage into the abscess was the cause of the early death." (*Dr. Conwell*, ibid, *p.* 517.)

No. 227.— ——, 3 years in India, in hospital 4 times in the previous 6 months, and on each occasion, treated with mercurials, admitted April 29th, 1831, with abdominal pain and muco-sanguineous stools. Symptoms. Pain in the back and nape of the neck, severe pain in the shoulders, easiest decubitus on the left side, burning at the epigastrium, prostration of strength, emaciation, vertigo, tongue and skin natural, pulse 74 to 104, soft, feeble, countenance like parchment, anorexia, restlessness. Latterly he had hectic fever with cold sweats, much cough and dyspnæa, great restlessness, occasional cramps in the lower extremities, hands and face puffed, not much derangement of the bowels. The urine is thus reported at several dates: May 16th, "urine copious, stained with bile,"—May 30th, "orange-coloured,"—June 30th, "dark,"—July 15th, "opaque and copious, like stale decoction of cinchona,"—July 31st, "opaque with pus,"—Aug. 15th, "like decoction of cinchona, with a little pus." He died September 3d.

Autopsy.—Liver congested; a large superficial abscess on the convex surface of the right lobe, which had burst, and discharged 5 pints of pus into the right thoracic cavity; the right lung was so closely compressed, and occupied such a small space, that at first sight it appeared to be altogether wanting; the hepatic tissue dark and carneous, containing few acini; extensive cerebral effusion; an abscess had formed under the chin, which was evacuated four days before death, but the sac was found re-filled with greenish-yellow pus. (*Dr. Conwell,* ibid, *p.* 519.)

No. 228.— ——, æt. 44, 28 years in India, tall, ruddy, of irregular habits, admitted with a fourth attack of hepatitis, Dec. 31st, 1831, having for ten days had pain, soreness, and uneasiness in the side and epigastrium; he had also oppression at the stomach, with nausea—pulse small and hard—skin cool and clammy—tongue red at the sides, foul in the centre—stools frequent, dark, sanguineous—urine very dark: he bore depletion badly, eight leeches causing sudden collapse. Mercury was given freely till Jan. 12th, when a tumour presented itself at the epigastrium; as this tumour became more prominent, *arterial pulsation in it was very distinct, although the patient was largely covered with bed-clothes;* he likewise suffered from palpitation of the heart. Subsequently there was much emaciation, debility, hectic fever, startings preventing sleep, a clammy state of the skin, and heat in the palms of the hands; pulse soft, small, and feeble, tongue red. Abscess opened Jan. 24th; he died Feb. 2d.

Autopsy.—Left lobe of the liver enlarged and firm, containing two large abscesses communicating with each other, and seventeen round white masses of fibro-cartilaginous tissue; right lobe natural; some pus had escaped through the artificial opening, into the abdominal cavity, giving rise to inflammation. The aorta, immediately above the cæliac artery, was encircled by a band of inflammation an inch broad, and the surrounding cellular tissue was injected with red gelatinized serum; this, as well as the pulsation in the tumour and the palpitation, was caused by the pressure of the left lobe. Case lxxviii in List of Operations. (*Dr. Conwell*, ibid, *p.* 521.)

No. 229.— ——, æt. 25, middle stature, fair, muscular, ill 2 years with rheumatism, for which he had been several times salivated; admitted Jan. 13th, with deranged bowels, great debility, œdema of the limbs, and an ulcer at the elbow; he suffered severely from rheumatic pains, and his left arm became partially paralytic; appetite good, stools nearly natural, pulse 120, large and soft, tongue pink and scarlet, urine at first clear, afterwards, opaque, purulent, and like decoction of cinchona. Died May 30th.

Autopsy.—Liver weighed 6¾ pounds; the right and left lobes were elongated downwards and forwards, and having embraced the gall-bladder completely, extended four inches below it on each side; thus the fundus of the gall-bladder presented itself on the anterior surface, four inches above the lower margin of the liver; this offered a yielding elastic prominence to the finger in the living body. Thirteen deep sulci were found on the convex surface, with extensive thickening and white corrugations covered with false membranes, and resembling scars; sections of these were smooth, shining, marbled, and of close structure; some patches retained the granular structure, others gradually changed to a close tissue, being pale or nearly white, and others were of a lardaceous consistence; some of them were semi-cartilaginous; a large branch of the hepatic vein ran from the two last mentioned spots, indicating probably the site of a former abscess (?); lobulus spigelii red and semi-cartilaginous; throughout the large intestines, and also in the cæcal extremity of the ilium, were chronic ulcerations; lungs healthy. (*Dr. Conwell*, ibid, *p.* 524.)

No. 230.— ——, æt. 41, 13 years in India, stout, healthy, prone to excesses, subject to hepatitis; admitted May 9th, 1832, after excessive drinking. The chief symptoms were pain in the right hypochondrium on turning or pressure, frequent vomiting and purging—stools at first muco-sanguineous, then red, mucous with dots of purulent matter, and lastly dark like coffee grounds—urine red, turbid, like ale, and passed with difficulty—skin dry, hot, and stinging, latterly clammy—much thirst—loss of appetite—restlessness—tongue heavily furred—pulse 116, soft.

Died May 16th. Treatment. Depletion, calomel, opium, ipecacuanha, blisters, &c.

Autopsy.—An abscess in the liver had opened into the ascending colon, in which was found some fluid like wine lees, with some flakes of pus; this had escaped from the abscess; the intestine and the hepatic tissue at the opening were in a sloughing state; right lobe adherent to the diaphragm. A large scar over the gall-bladder, of which the centre formed a broad deep notch or fissure; the mucous coat of stomach, duodenum, and ilium, with traces of congestion; colon and cæcum filled with numerous ulcers, some in a sloughing state; lungs congested. (*Dr. Conwell,* ibid, *p.* 526.)

No. 231.—W. T., æt. 30, ill 7 days with dysentery, admitted Aug. 10th; ascribes this attack to a severe fall, which caused intense pain in the right side, which remained on admission; he had also pain on pressure in the hypogastric region, frequent bilious stools with slime, and tenesmus; headache, intense thirst, restlessness, and loss of appetite; tongue furred and dry; skin hot and feverish; pulse full and rapid. These symptoms, though relieved by V. S., leeches, calomel, opium, &c., continued till the 13th, when he became delirious; the pulse also became small and feeble, skin relaxed, abdomen tense and rather tender. Vomiting of bilious matter, hiccup, and involuntarily passing muco-sanguineous stools, preceded death on the 17th.

Autopsy.—Liver enlarged, of granular structure, with two large abscesses in the right lobe, one of which had burst and discharged its contents (pure pus) into the abdomen—abscess-walls had a ragged appearance—gall-bladder small, distended with thick, black, tar-like bile—cæcum and colon covered with sloughing gangrenous ulcers, on the surface of which small coagula of blood were observed—spleen and kidneys healthy—lungs congested—brain congested and indurated, with effusion into the ventricles—hypertrophy of the right ventricle of the heart. (*Mr. Roosmaleecoq, in Webb's Pathologia Indica, p. 272.*)

No. 232.—James, æt. 30, Englishman, cachectic, intemperate; a year before in hospital with syphilis; admitted Aug. 9th, 1847, with an indolent ulcer on the left leg; whilst this was healing under a slight mercurial course, dysentery supervened. On Sept. 16th, he complained, for the first time, of pain on pressure

Note.—Dr. Conwell's 17th case of hepatic abscess (No. 232 of his cases,) has been purposely omitted; the dissection report affords no evidence of abscess; the white scar, may have arisen from some other cause than the bursting of an abscess.

about the umbilicus; skin hot and dry; pulse small and rapid; stools solid. Subsequently a *tumour presented itself about the umbilicus, in which there was distinct pulsation, as if it were proceeding from an aneurism;* this was absent when the patient bent forward; the tumour assumed a conical form, and was tender to the touch; on Oct. 1st, there was distinct fluctuation, and on the 2d, the abscess apparently burst, as the abdomen became quite even and soft; he became extremely weak; had cold clammy perspirations, and died Oct. 3d. At no period was there pain in the shoulder.

Autopsy.—Liver enlarged and congested; in the lower part of the posterior surface of the liver was a large abscess, which had burst and discharged about 2 pints of pus into the abdominal cavity; the intestines agglutinated together; coats of the colon thickened; no mention of ulceration; no other organic lesion observable. (*Mr. Loftus, in Webb's Path. Indica, p. 274.*)

No. 233.—Gunner, æt. 25, bowels deranged some months, admitted Aug. 26th, 1845, with constipation and slight fever. Except weakness and a yellow suffusion of the skin, no signs of hepatic disease evidenced themselves till Sept. 14th, when he complained for the first time of pain in the right iliac region; on the 16th, there was some tension at the head of the right rectus muscle, and the liver was observed to project below the margin of the ribs; on the 17th, he had a rigor. The other symptoms were distention of the abdomen, much flatus, great weakness, disturbed rest, an extremely suffused state of the skin, and exhaustion; stools healthy or dark-green; urine copious, and surcharged with bile; pulse rapid, soft, intermittent at times; tongue brown and dry. Slight delirium preceded death, on Oct. 5th. Treatment. Mercury, purgatives, &c., early in the disease.

Autopsy.—Liver slightly enlarged, very firm, of a compressed and rounded form, contained two abscesses; one small on the superior surface of the right lobe, full of thick purulent matter, deeply tinged with bile, and lined with a smooth membrane; the second, with 5 or 6 ounces of pus in it, was on the under surface of the right lobe, and was lined with a thick membranous exudation; it had formed a communication with the cellular tissue surrounding the right kidney; it had also formed adhesions to the duodenum. Gall-bladder large, containing dark, tenacious bile. The hepatic and other ducts quite pervious; *an opening was found, by which the abscess communicated with the hepatic vein, at its junction with the vena cava.* (*Dr. Clark, in Webb's Path. Indica, p. 276.*)

No. 234.—Ummer Doss, admitted Aug. 1st, 1841, bowels not open for 7 days. A swelling, with an elastic feel, about the size of a closed fist, existed under the margin of the ribs on the right side; it was neither red, hot nor tender; had been there five days—belly as hard as a board—little pain—vomiting of food—tongue red and broad—pulse very weak. On the 5th, the swelling was larger; a little manipulation was used, as it was thought to be a knot of the intestine; gentle pressure on it caused it to disappear; the reduction was followed by much pain. Up to the 10th, he had passed no proper stool—the belly remained as hard as a board—he had much abdominal pain, and great thirst—tongue smooth, red, and dry, with elongated papillæ protruding from it. He became a mere skeleton, and died on the 12th. Treatment. Leeches, strong purgatives, enemas, &c.

Autopsy.—Liver adherent to the stomach, and to all the contiguous surfaces; intestines matted together, their mucous coat entire; the whole bowel seemed softened or rotten; in the right lobe of the liver was a superficial abscess, filled with thick pus, intimately adherent to the colon; a second abscess, having thick walls of coagulable lymph, existed between the upper convex surface of the right lobe and the diaphragm, filled with sero-purulent matter mixed with albuminous flakes. *The hepatic veins appeared to contain pus.* Anus obstructed by piles; an abscess in perinæo. N. B. The swelling above described was probably a fold of intestine, adhering to the abscess on one side, and to the walls of the abdomen on the other, as a gurgling sound was heard upon its retrocession. (*Dr. Allan Webb, Path. Indica, p.* 278.)

No. 235.—J. Smith, æt. 27, admitted July 24th, with severe dysentery and excruciating abdominal pain. Under the use of V. S., blue pill, opium, and ipecacuanha, the dysenteric symptoms subsided in a great measure, and on the 11th, he was seized with acute hepatic pain, which yielded to leeches, blisters, &c. Latterly he had no uneasiness about the liver, the stools contained no blood; the tongue blanched, the forehead bathed in perspiration, pulse small. He gradually sank, and died Aug. 28th.

Autopsy.—In the right lobe of the liver was a huge encysted abscess, large enough to contain a man's head, the cyst lined by albuminous and fibrinous concretions; the enormous distention of the structure strengthened by adhesions to the surrounding parts; left lobe sound; the mucous coat of the colon presented small granular points, but there was little appearance of inflammation or its effects. (*Dr. W. C. McGregor, in Webb's Pathologia Indica, p.* 280.)

No. 236.—An old resident in Bengal, a hard liver, ill for some months with hepatic disease; admitted with much fulness of the right side, cough, and slight pyrexia; but the disease was too far advanced for active treatment. In about a week after admission, he began to expectorate, and suddenly brought up a pint of matter from the lungs. Treatment not given.

Autopsy.—The abscess apparently commenced on the most convex part of the liver, not implicating much the organ; it had burst into the chest through the diaphragm, forming with the lungs one large cavity. The extent of disorganization was very great, "large blood vessels, disorganized tissues, and the wreck of the air passages and pulmonary structure, were all confounded together in one gaping ruin." (*Dr. Jackson, in Webb's Path. Indica, p. 282.*)

No. 237.—M. Sheild, æt. 21, ill 9 weeks with dysentery and fever. The dysenteric symptoms were so severe as to mask, in a great measure, the signs of hepatic disease; there was no pain on pressure on any part of the abdomen except over the cæcum, and then only slightly, two days before death; and there do not appear to have been rigors, vomiting or pain in the shoulder. Latterly the stools, from being dysenteric, became brown and feculent with dark bile, and on the day of death (Oct. 20th) they consisted of black fluid, without blood or mucus. Treatment. V.S., blue pill, quinine, ipecacuanha, &c.

Autopsy.—Liver of healthy appearance; in the right lobe were four small abscesses, each containing half an ounce of pus; gall-bladder nearly empty. In the cæcum and colon numerous ulcerations, with much vascularity and thickening of the coats; small intestines and stomach healthy; some of the mesenteric glands were enlarged, and in the centre of one was about a drachm of thick pus. (*H. Bedborough, Esq., in Webb's Path. Indica, p. 284.*)

No. 238.—H. Crawford, a recruit, æt. 21, temperate, very delicate, admitted Nov. 1st, 1842, with dysentery. On the 9th, he complained, for the first time, of pain in the epigastric region; there was also tenseness of the abdominal muscles; next day there was a swelling in the right side, a little below the margin of the false ribs; this tumour continued to increase and become more prominent, till the 13th, when it appeared less in size and softer, but the pain on pressure remained undiminished; the tumour now became smaller and less painful on pressure, till the period of his death. The other symptoms were, emaciation, prostration, occasional vomiting, hiccup and restlessness; pulse small, frequent; tongue red, coated in the centre; countenance sunken; purgatives appear to have been necessary to keep the bowels open. He died

Nov. 18th. Calomel was only given occasionally as a purgative; other treatment palliative.

Autopsy.—A large abscess in the left lobe of the liver, firmly adherent to the ribs; general peritoneal inflammation; lungs healthy in structure. (*W. Craigie, Esq., in Webb's Path. Indica, p. 285.*)

No. 239.—J. Cunningham, ill several months, admitted Nov. 9th, 1852, with hepatic abscess in an advanced state; there was fulness and tension of the right side, occasional pain in the liver, œdema of the legs—tongue foul—pulse frequent and soft—appetite good—bowels free—motions feculent; on Nov. 19th, the abscess apparently burst into the abdominal cavity, as intense peritonitis set in, with fulness, tension, and pain in the abdomen, &c. He became gradually worse; the abdomen was distended, hard, and tender, and he had urgent thirst, great anxiety and distress, and constant moaning. He died Nov. 24th. The early treatment not given.

Autopsy.—Liver enlarged; in the right lobe a large abscess which had burst into the abdominal cavity, and discharged much sero-purulent matter. The abscess was adherent to the colon, but no communication between the cavity and the intestine could be traced; mucous coat of intestines vascular in places; general peritoneal inflammation; spleen enlarged; lungs not diseased. (*Dr. J. Sutherland, in Webb's Path. Indica, p. 287.*)

No. 240.—P. Pitten, English sailor, æt. 33, admitted Nov. 4th, with acute pain in the left lobe of the liver, increased on pressure; right lobe not tender, but seemed rather full; abdomen very hot and tense—nausea, inability to lie easily on the left side—no pain in the shoulders—tongue brown—skin hot—pulse quick and full—bowels regular; the symptoms were well marked, and were treated with mercury externally and internally, leeches, blisters, &c. These had apparently good effect; on the 13th, the report is, "no fulness of the side, is able to lie on any side without any inconvenience, bowels regular, tongue clean, skin cool, pulse natural." On the 14th, he was discharged at his own request. *Re-admitted Nov. 20th*, with loss of motion of the right arm and leg, head hot, and pupils contracted; on protruding his tongue, it inclined to the right side. These symptoms came on four days previously, and consequently two days after his discharge; the subsequent symptoms were those of the cerebral affection; he became comatose, urine and feces were passed involuntarily, and he died on the 28th.

Autopsy.—*Head;* sub-arachnoid effusion, great congestion of the pia mater, substance of the left hemisphere of the brain congested and softened, and in its centre was an abscess containing an ounce of well digested pus. The right hemisphere firmer than natural, deeply injected in its white substance. *Spinal marrow* softened in its centre. *Heart;* substance generally inflamed and softened, the pericardiac covering thickened by opacities, encordia of both auricles opaque; in the right ventricle an organized coagulum prolonged into the pulmonary artery. *Liver*, enlarged, softened, and congested, with whitish maculæ or striæ; soft and rapidly wrinkling by exposure to the air; adherent to the diaphragm; contained four abscesses, two in the right lobe, one in the left, and one in the middle lobe, encysted, full of pus. Stomach and intestines healthy; kidneys congested; spleen healthy. (*Dr. Jackson, in Webb's Path. Indica, p. 288.*)

No. 241.—C. Harrington, sailor, æt. 33, ill 6 days with hepatitis; admitted Oct. 8th, with pain and fulness in the epigastrium and right hypochondrium; also *pain in the left shoulder*, none in the right—inability to lie on the left side—abdomen tense and resisting—urine scanty and high coloured—bowels costive—pulse rather full—tongue yellow in the centre. The remedies used afforded little relief, and on the 12th, he had much pain in the left side, extending from the hypochondrium to the shoulder; the other symptoms were tension of the right rectus muscle, occasional vomiting, startings in the sleep at nights, and profuse sweats—countenance anxious—pulse rapid, feeble—stools watery—tongue morbidly red at the tip, brownish in the centre, and glazed. Fluctuation being evident, the abscess was opened on the 28th; he died two days after.

Autopsy.—Liver contained three abscesses, one in the right lobe adherent to the false ribs, had been evacuated by operation; the second had opened into the duodenum, just below the pylorus, immediately to the left of the gall-bladder, to which last the duodenum was firmly adherent; the third abscess was in the left lobe; it extended upward towards the diaphragm which it had perforated, and then taking a downward course, it had opened into the stomach, about three inches below its cardiac orifice, through an ulcerated opening. Kidneys slightly diseased; heart somewhat enlarged, on its surface some flakes of coagulable lymph. Case lxxix in List of Operations. (*Dr. Jackson*, ibid, *p.* 290.)

No. 242.—J. Russel, æt. 24, 3 years in India, fair complexion, admitted Dec. 9th, 1843, with intermittent fever; on the 14th, he had acute pain in the left boundary of the epigastrium and left hypochondrium, increased by full inspiration; and on the

16th, there was distinct fulness in the left hypochondrium, extending to the sternum; percussion gave a dull sound, indicating enlargement of the left lobe of the liver; decubitus easiest on the right side; no rigors; pulse 69, soft, weak; tongue moist; much perspiration. Mercury was given freely, and slight ptyalism established; urine for some time had a copious white deposit, and subsequently was turbid without deposit. He had latterly hectic with night sweats, and emaciation; fluctuation being evident the abscess was opened, with temporary relief; but hectic progressed, delirium set in, and he died Jan. 11th. Amongst other measures a seton was inserted, and an incision made over the tumour down to the peritoneum.

Autopsy.—Left lobe of the liver extremely enlarged, adherent to the abdominal parietes, stomach, and spleen. The abscess occupied nearly the whole of the left side of the organ, and contained a large quantity of matter mixed with sloughy shreds; the substance of the liver round it, was soft, and gave way easily on pressure; the right lobe also enlarged with abscesses, few larger than hazel nuts, scattered throughout; around them was no inflammatory appearance; in some the matter was as thick as curd. All the other abdominal and thoracic viscera healthy. Case lxxxi in List of Operations. (*Dr. F. Anderson, in Webb's Path. Ind. p.* 120.)

No. 243.—G. Chumley, admitted with delirium tremens, Oct. 31st; died of disease of the liver, Nov. 30th, 1846. History not given.

Autopsy.—Right lobe of the liver studded with small abscesses; left lobe occupied by a large abscess, which communicated with the stomach. (*Mr. Loftus, in Webb's Path. Indica, p.* 262.)

No. 244.—A girl, about 16 years old, at the Orphan School Hospital in Calcutta, under the care of Mr. Egerton; she had seven abscesses in the course of an attack of fever; one in the elbow, one in the arm, one on each leg, one in the thigh, and one large one in the liver; the latter burst by sloughing, opening backwards through the ribs of the back. When the abdomen was pressed, large quantities of matter came out behind. On opening the body, the sac was found in a sloughing state. (*Webb's Path. Indica, p.* 112.)

No. 245.—S. Maisey, ill 14 days with dysentery, admittted Sept. 3d, 1845; a fulness over the hepatic region, without any pain, indicated suppuration. He died Sept. 29th.

Autopsy.—Nearly the entire of the right lobe of the liver formed a sacculated abscess, containing 3 pounds of thick purulent matter; gall-bladder distended with thick grumous bile; colon vascular throughout, with spots of ulceration; stomach vascular, containing much green, bilious fluid; spleen and kidneys natural; right lung atrophied. (*Dr. Mouat, in Webb's Pathologia Indica, p.* 260.)

No. 246.—S. Shaw, æt. 24, admitted May 29th; abscess opened Oct. 21st; died Nov. 2d. There was copious expectoration of muco-purulent matter. History of the case not given.

Autopsy.—Liver adherent firmly to the diaphragm and side; in the right lobe were two abscesses, each containing 4 ounces of pus; in the one which had been punctured was a quantity of pure looking bile; gall-bladder empty. In the edge of the left lobe was a small superficial abscess; colon contracted, ulcerated, some of the ulcers healing; other organs healthy; right lung hepatized and shrunk; body much emaciated. Case lvii in List of Operations. (*Madras Medical Journal,* vol. vi, *p.* 331.)

No. 247.—C. Hopkins, æt. 22, admitted with hepatic dysentery, Nov. 12th, 1841; abscess opened Dec. 12th; died on the 16th. History not given.

Autopsy.—A large abscess in the right lobe of the liver, the sac partially emptied of its contents by operation; ulceration in the arch of and in the descending colon; heart normal; other organs healthy. Case liii in List of Operations. (*Dr. Dempster, Mad. Med. Journal,* vol. vi.)

No. 248.—T. Darknell, æt. 28, admitted Sept. 15th, 1843; abscess opened Oct. 21st; died Nov. 5th. Not combined with dysentery. Symptoms not given.

Autopsy.—Liver large, studded with small abscesses; in the right lobe one large abscess containing 2 pounds of sero-purulent matter; left lobe tolerably healthy—gall-bladder distended and enlarged—stomach and intestines healthy throughout, but contracted, especially the stomach, which was not larger than the duodenum—contents of head and thorax healthy—kidneys normal—body emaciated. Case lii in List of Operations. (*J. P. Grant, Esq.,* ibid, vol. vi, *p.* 329.)

No. 249.—W. Quinlow, æt. 27, admitted April 21st, died Aug. 8th; abscess opened; history of the case not given.

Autopsy.—Liver not much altered in size; the right lobe thickly studded with abscesses, varying in size from a pea upwards; the abscess opened was mid-way between the right and left lobes, capable of holding 12 ounces; its walls were composed of dense parenchymatous tissue, and the surface was honey-combed; intestines pale and healthy; in the lower fifth of the ilium were numerous ulcers about an inch in diameter, with thickened and everted edges; also a number of small abscesses about the cæcum coli; the walls slightly thickened. Lungs and heart healthy—about one pound of clear serum in the pericardium. Case lvi in List of Operations. (*Mad. Med. Journ.* vol. vi, *p.* 331.)

No. 250.—J. McGill, æt. 25, admitted Dec. 29th, 1841, died April 2d, 1842. Abscess opened; not combined with dysentery; history not given.

Autopsy.—In the liver were two abscesses; one large superficial, containing 12 ounces of pus, in the outer part of the right lobe; (this had been opened;) and the second, the size of a goose's egg, was on the under surface of the left lobe. Case xliv in List of Operations. (*Ibid*, vol. vi, *p.* 326.)

No. 251.—J. Macdonald, æt. 25, admitted May 2d, 1841, died July 29th, 4 days after the abscess had been opened: combined with dysentery—history of the case not given.

Autopsy.—Liver firmly adherent to the side, and also to the colon; it contained only one abscess, the one punctured; its walls had no distinct capsule, its boundary being uneven, and formed by the irregularly excavated substance of the liver, which was soft and dark; the abscess contained several ounces of dark, yellow, offensive matter; colon extensively but not deeply ulcerated; its mucous coat surrounding the ulcers softened, tumid, and of a dark-red colour—thoracic viscera healthy—body emaciated. Case lv in List of Operations. (*Dr. J. Anderson*, ibid, *p.* 333.)

No. 252.—J. Wake, æt. 26, admitted with hepatitis May 5th, 1842, abscess opened May 31st, discharged Aug. 22d, re-admitted Nov. 6th, died Nov. 12th. Symptoms and treatment not given.

Autopsy.—Liver much diseased; two large and several small abscesses in the right lobe, and one in the left; their contents flaky, purulent, of a pale yellow colour. The liver was enveloped in adhesions, in which the colon, stomach, and spleen were included; the lower surface of the left lobe was much ulcerated, and a large quantity of pus was enclosed by adhesions existing between it and the stomach. Case xlvi in List of Operations. (*Dr. Thompson*, ibid, vol. vi, *p.* 327.)

No. 253.—W. Morris, H. M. 4th Regt., sunk under the formation of an extensive abscess of the liver, extending downwards, and completely destroying the right kidney. In the left lobe were several hard, large, white, tubercular masses. (*Dr. Sievwright, Madras Medical Journal*, vol. i, *p.* 138.)

No. 254.—Mrs. Longsworth, a fine young woman, but intemperate; much hurt in a scuffle 14 days before admission; from that time she suffered much from pain in the right side. On admission the right hypochondrium was tumified, and extremely tender on pressure; the swelling subsequently became more prominent, and gave an obscure feeling of fluctuation; dyspnæa urgent; diarrhœa and hectic set in, and she died 38 days after admission.

Autopsy.—A large superficial abscess in the right lobe of the liver; it was near the surface, and firmly adherent to the side. An operation would probably have saved her life, but she declined having it performed. (*Dr. Henderson*, ibid, vol. iii, *p.* 151.)

No. 255.—J. McEldoon, æt. 38, 12 years in India, healthy, lately intemperate; admitted Nov. 10th, 1839, with severe pain in the right hypochondrium, increased by inspiration on pressure—ill three days—he also had severe headache. Subsequently the liver became enlarged, extending into the epigastrium, very tender to the touch, and latterly fluctuation was perceptible. Gums sore and ulcerated, but without ptyalism, though mercury was given freely; cold sweats, emaciation, a sense of weight and oppression in the epigastrium, were present; bowels open, motions dark-green. Abscess opened, matter evacuated; he partially recovered, was sent to England, and died on the passage, 6 months after the operation.

Autopsy—Given fully in Case vii in List of Operations. The liver was a little larger than natural—site of the abscess not ascertained—small intestines vascular—the large ones, particularly the rectum, covered with patches of ulceration, and studded with spots of old ulcers, which had healed up. (*Drs. Everard and Mockler, Madras Med. Journal,* vol. ii, *p.* 299, and vol. iii, *p.* 392.)

No. 256.—Andiappen, a native (?) æt. 37, admitted April 27th, died May 28th, 1843; 29 days after the abscess had been opened. History of the case not given.

Autopsy.—Right lobe of the liver much enlarged and dark; the abscess opened, was on the anterior border of the liver; its walls black and sloughy; posteriorly it communicated with a deeper and larger sac, filled with thick curdy matter; the walls of this likewise were dark and sloughy, with a most offensive odour. Case xlviii in List of Operations. (*J. Shaw, Esq.*, ibid, vol. vi, *p.* 324.

No. 257.—G. E., æt. 34, admitted Dec. 2d; died Dec. 28th, 1843, the day after the evacuation of the abscess. History of the case not given.

Autopsy.—The right lobe of the liver much enlarged; the abscess occupied nearly the whole lobe, and was filled with thin curdy pus; cyst adherent to the side. Case l in List of Operations. (*James Shaw, Esq.*, ibid.)

No. 258.—Jackson, æt. 34, admitted March 19th; died April 20th. The immediate cause of death was hæmorrhage into the sac of the abscess, after the evacuation of the abscess. Symptoms not given.

Autopsy.—Liver enlarged, extending as high as the 4th rib; the right lobe was the mere sac of an abscess, and contained a large quantity of purulent matter, with several coagula of blood; hæmorrhage had taken place from a small vessel at the floor of the abscess, near the transverse fissure; left lobe of a tawny colour, and easily broken down. There were old adhesions at the caput coli, binding it down to the brim of the pelvis; in the cæcum were some ulcers, apparently of old standing. Case xlix in List of Operations. (*James Shaw, Esq.*, ibid, *p.* 325.)

No. 259.—J. Belincoe, æt. 30, admitted Oct. 19th; abscess opened; died Nov. 18th, 1842, 15 days after operation. History not given.

Autopsy.—Liver much enlarged; in the left lobe one large abscess, which was making its way by ulcerative inflammation through the coats of the stomach; right lobe studded with yellow patches. Case xlv in List of Operations. (*Madras Medical Journal*, vol. vi, *p.* 327.)

No. 260.—Capt. H., admitted Dec. 3d; died Jan. 6th, 1841, 5 days after the abscess had been opened. History not given.

Autopsy.—In the liver were five abscesses; one of them contained between 4 and 5 pints of purulent matter. Case liv in List of Operations. (*Dr. Anderson*, ibid, vol. vi, *p.* 332.)

No. 261.—J. Wells, æt. 36, admitted June 26th, died Aug. 2d, 1842, 14 days after the abscess had been opened. Combined with diarrhoea. History not given. Case lviii in List of Operations.

Autopsy.—Liver enormously enlarged; the right lobe formed the cyst of one large abscess containing 3 pints of very thick pus; the abscess communicated through the diaphragm with the right lung; adhesions to the side; left lobe healthy. (*Madras Medical Journal*, vol. vi, *p.* 331.)

No. 262.—A man died in hospital at Meerut, who had been subject for three years to attacks of hepatitis. The first had been severe, but latterly he used to be 10 or 14 days in hospital at different times, with a pain in the side and shoulder, which would then leave him; in the last attack he had similar symptoms, and an abscess burst into the peritoneum, the third day after admission. (*Dr. Murray*, ibid, vol. i, *p.* 175.)

No. 263.—Dr. Wilkinson, of H. M. 22d Regt. He first had all the symptoms of dysentery, which subsided, under what treatment is not stated; then anomalous symptoms came on with excitement, under which suppuration in the liver formed. The dissection showed that a small abscess had burst into the abdomen, yet the intestines were all sound. (*Dr. McDonell*, ibid, vol. ii, *p.* 40.)

No. 264 and 265.—Two men in H. M. 57th Regt., treated for acute hepatitis, died in 1838. In each of these two fatal cases, in addition to a large abscess in the right lobe of the liver, there was ulceration and sloughing of the mucous coat of the large intestine, from the cæcal valve to the anus. (*Dr. A. B. Morgan*, ibid, vol. ii, *p.* 135.)

No. 266.—A soldier in H. M. 39th Regt., admitted with hepatitis, and died at Poonamallee in 1832. He was a man of decidedly scrofulous habit, and on dissection the liver was found to be one continuous abscess. (*Dr. Hamilton*, ibid, vol. ii, *p.* 244.)

No. 267.—A striking instance of the insidious character of hepatic abscess. A soldier in H. M. 55th Regt., died at Secunderabad, in 1839. *An abscess had burst into the lungs when at his duty*, and he was expectorating large quantities of blood and pus when admitted into hospital. (*Dr. Shanks*, ibid, vol. iii, *p.* 29.)

No. 268.—S. Cox, H. M. 41st Regt., admitted with continued fever at Moulmein; and died in 1832. History of the case not given.

Autopsy.—Abscess in the liver, colon ulcerated, spleen soft, lungs congested, nothing remarkable in the head. (*Dr. Hamilton*, ibid, vol. iii, *p.* 208.)

No. 269.—T. Davies, H. M. 41st Regt., admitted with continued fever. The history of the case is not given. Dissection showed the liver enlarged, and containing a collection of pus; there were extensive adhesions in the thorax, but nothing remarkable in the head. (*Dr. Hamilton*, ibid.)

No. 270.—J. Keough, H. M. 41st Regt., admitted with dysentery, which proved fatal. Dissection disclosed an abscess in the liver, and an ulcerated state of the colon. (*Dr. Hamilton*, ibid.)

No. 271.—A soldier, in H. M. 41st Regt., admitted with hepatitis in 1832. The inflammation terminated on two successive occasions in abscess, the contents of which found an outlet, in the first attack by the bowels, and in the second by the mouth. Tonics, &c., were given, but he ultimately sank. On dissection no communication with either the intestines or stomach and the liver could be detected, to explain in what manner the diseased fluid had become successively thrown off by these outlets. (*Dr. Hamilton*, ibid, vol. iii, *p.* 214.)

No. 272.—Sergeant Lees, admitted with hepatitis, which terminated in suppuration. The abscess burst into the lungs, and for a considerable period he coughed up about a pint of matter daily. He ultimately sank under diarrhœa and hectic.

Autopsy.—The whole of the upper part of the right lobe of the liver, disorganized; the diaphragm had given way; the lower part of the right lung highly diseased, and connected firmly to the remaining portion of the diaphragm; the whole forming, with the aid of the pleura costalis, the walls of an immense abscess. (*Dr. Henderson*, ibid, vol. iii, *p.* 313.)

No. 273.—A soldier, in H. M. 4th Regt., admitted with hepatitis, which terminated in abscess. History of the case not given.

Autopsy.—In the right lobe of the liver was found a very large abscess, which contained two pints of pus. State of the intestines not noticed. (*Dr. W. Milligan*, ibid, vol. iv, *p.* 112.)

No. 274.—W. Gittus, æt. 35, 10 years in India, sanguine temperament, admitted with acute hepatitis, Nov. 12th, 1834. The urgent symptoms yielded to mercurials, leeches, &c., but he continued emaciated and delicate up to Dec. 17th, when he complained of pain in the liver, extending to both shoulders; and on the 24th, he expectorated bloody purulent matter, which increased daily in quantity, often amounting to 4 pounds in 24 hours. He continued in this state up to Feb. 7th, when he complained of pain in his left great toe, and a blueish spot, the size of a sixpence was perceived on the ball, and another spot at the inner ankle; the instep soon became tumid, and an erysipelatous redness with some hardness was traced along the inner and back part of the leg, following the course of the lymphatics and blood vessels, from the ham to the groin; the expectoration of pus began to diminish, and ceased altogether on the 8th of February. The swelling of the limb rapidly increased, and the surface of the foot and toes was of a dark livid colour; pain was only felt on the instep from distention, the dark colour quickly extended over the whole limb—partial clammy sweating—features anxious but mind calm. On the 8th, the limb was twice the size of the other, and the swelling did not extend beyond Poupart's ligament; the foot retained its natural heat, and the pain was always referred to the instep. On the 9th, the lividity of the limb was general, and the surface shining—slightly pitting on pressure.

Emaciation now became very rapid, and on the 11th, the swelling of the limb began to subside, and the colour of the surface appeared more natural. On the 12th, a blister, which had formed at the inner ankle burst, and discharged serum; the mind began to wander, and weakness increased. The sore near the ankle enlarged, but not gangrenous, extremities cold; he became perfectly fatuous; swelling of the limb nearly disappeared, and he sank Feb. 22d.

Post-mortem.—The foot alone was swollen and œdematous; surface of the limb of dull colour; an infiltration of serum beneath the cutis, and *the veins of the limb thickened and inflamed from the foot to the groin, and filled with coagula;* the femoral vein very much enlarged at the groin. The right lung was injected with a thin bloody fluid; bronchial tubes dilated, and the lining membrane of the trachea and bronchi of a deep-red colour, and covered with unhealthy looking mucus. Strong adhesions existed between the lower lobe of the lung and the floor of the diaphragm, through which a communication was established with the upper and convex surface of the liver, which contained a large abscess full of pus. (*Selections from the Reports of H. M. 39th Regt. in Madras Medical Journal*, vol. iv, *p.* 347.)

No. 275.—J. Burton, æt. 34, admitted with common continued fever; whilst under treatment for this, a sudden diversion took place to the liver, and notwithstanding V. S., leeches, and the use of mercury, an abscess formed—fluctuation obscure—abscess opened,—lived eight days after, and then sank from exhaustion. Case xxxviii in List of Operations.

Autopsy.—Liver adherent to the side; the position or number of the abscesses not given. (*Dr. Dix*, ibid, vol. v, *p.* 212.)

No. 276 and 277.—Two soldiers, in H. M. 4th Regt., died in 1842, of hepatitis. In both the hepatic affection was complicated with severe dysenteric symptoms; and in both, in addition to an enormous abscess in the right lobe of the liver, the colon exhibited through its whole course, extensive traces of disorganization. (*Dr. Parry*, ibid, vol. v, *p.* 322.)

No. 278.—A soldier, in H. M. 4th Regt., died of abscess in the liver, supervening upon hepatitis. On dissection, the liver was found to contain a plurality of abscesses, 3 in the right, and 2 in the left lobe. (*Dr. Parry*, ibid.)

No. 279.—W. Linnett, æt. 30, 5 years in India, admitted with a third attack of dysentery, under which he sank in 12 days. There was tendernesss of the abdomen, with muco-sanguineous stools and dysuria. He was bled and leeched, but it does not appear that he took mercury.

Autopsy.—The liver contained four abscesses; large intestines ulcerated. (*Dr. Innis*, ibid, vol. vi, *p.* 169.)

No. 280.—M. Callagahan, æt. 25, 4½ years in India, admitted with a relapse of dysentery—duration of the disease 11 days. In addition to the dysenteric stools, he had tenderness of the abdomen, and dysuria. Blood-letting, ipecacuanha, and opium formed the main treatment.

Autopsy.—The liver contained numerous abscesses; the large intestines ulcerated, and in parts perforated. (*Dr. Innis.*)

No. 281.—P. Barrow, æt. 33, 5½ years in India, admitted with dysentery, which was treated by V. S., ipecac, and opium. He died on the 8th day. The symptoms were chiefly dysenteric.

Autopsy.—Large intestines ulcerated—liver contained four abscesses. (*Dr. Innis.*)

No. 282.—T. Young, æt. 30, 5½ years in India, admitted with dysentery, which proved fatal in 30 days. Leeches, ipecac, and opium formed the main treatment.

Autopsy.—Large intestines ulcerated, and in the liver were found three abscesses. (*Dr. Innis.*)

No. 283.—J. Caddigan, æt. 35, 6 years in India, admitted with dysentery, which proved fatal on the 25th day. In addition to dysenteric symptoms, he had dysuria; he does not appear to have taken mercury.

Autopsy.—Large intestines ulcerated. There was a large abscess, containing two quarts of pus, between the convex surface of the liver and the diaphragm; it had burst into the cavity of the pleura. After death, three punctures were made into the liver, and not one of them reached the abscess. (*Dr. Innis.*)

No. 284.—An Artilleryman in the Bombay Service. The particulars of the case not given. Abscess formed, and the tumefaction in the side gradually disappeared. After death, *the abscess was found nearly empty, and two hepatic ducts communicating with it, were found carrying pus to the duodenum.* (*Mr. Leith, Trans. of the Med. and Phys. Society of Bombay*, No. iv, *p.* 57.)

No. 285.—A Sailor, æt. 63, admitted with hepatitis. The symptoms were badly marked; there was constant depression of spirits, frequent moaning, oppressed pulse,—little complaint of pain, which was confined to the right hypochondrium, till the day before death, when he had excruciating pain in the abdomen (from the bursting of the abscess?). Duration of the disease 20 days.

Autopsy.—Sero-purulent effusion into the abdominal cavity, and the whole of the peritoneal coat of the intestines was bright-red and coated with flakes of pus. A superficial abscess was found in the liver. (*Dr. J. Bird*, ibid, vol. ii, *p.* 60.)

No. 286.—A Hindoo, treated in the General Hospital in Calcutta. No history given. An abscess had formed in the convex surface of the right lobe, ulcerating through the diaphragm, and had emptied its contents into the right thorax. Fibrinous dropsy ensued, coating with plastic layers the whole of the lung, which was reduced to the size of a closed hand; the heart small, and its parietes very thin. The weight of the superincumbent fluid had pressed down *the liver, till it was as flat throughout as a hand, and scarcely exceeding a hand in size.* (*Webb's Path. Indica, p.* 262.)

No. 287.—A Native woman, æt. 30. History not given. On dissection, many little abscesses were found in the right lobe, and one large one at its anterior extremity, which had become adherent to the transverse colon; there was another abscess of similar size in the middle of the left lobe, which part was adherent to the right kidney. The other organs seemed healthy. The abscesses were non-encysted. (*Webb*, ibid, *p.* 262.)

No. 288.—T. A., æt. 21, a stout, pale, robust youth, seized in August with diarrhœa, which continued for some weeks, in spite of all treatment; he also complained of rheumatic (?) pains in the extremities, and of a dull pain in the right hypochondrium. In September, in consequence of exposure during convalescence, he was seized with a violent intermittent fever, which continued for a month, although quinine was administered freely. His constitution became much impaired, and although he improved, there were still hectic flushes, and occasional cold sweats. After again exposing himself imprudently, he was attacked with a severe pain in the bowels, slight cough, and pain in the right side —followed next day by the most severe spasms, and difficulty of breathing, a strong, full, bounding pulse, high fever, and incessant cough. He was treated as actively as his emaciated condition would admit; the cough however daily increased, and in November, the expectoration was copious and purulent, with increase of hectic fever. He was now extremely feeble, and in an endeavour to turn round in bed, *he fractured the femur in an oblique direction;* all attempts to produce union failed. The purulent expectoration continued, and he sank in the beginning of December.

Autopsy.—Strong adhesions between the liver and diaphragm; the lung was also firmly adherent to the upper surface of the diaphragm, and on examination, all appearance of that muscle was found obliterated, except a narrow border, by which it maintained its position to the narrow walls of the great cavity. In the centre of the liver were found 5 or 6 large cavities filled with pus; from these there proceeded several sinuses, passing through what had formed the diaphragm, extending through the substance of the right lung, and opening into the bronchial ramifications, in which there was found a considerable quantity of pus. One of these sinuses was so large as to admit of the little finger. The lung was much consolidated, but otherwise healthy. The heart and arteries, the alimentary canal, the spleen and kidneys, were all natural, except that the latter were paler than usual, and the heart somewhat attenuated. On examining the fracture, the bone was found in a state of caries; so soft, that parts of it could be rubbed to powder between the thumb and finger—periosteum separated, but there was no appearance of suppuration. (*A. Webb*, ibid, *p*. 126.)

No. 289.—W. Green, æt. 38, sailor, tall, large, of dark complexion, recently from England—admitted with severe dysentery—ill 14 days. He was much reduced; belly flat, inelastic, and tender if pressed; pyrexia moderate; pulse from 96 to 116. Died 52 hours after admission.

Autopsy.—Liver slightly enlarged, pale, soft, unctuous; in its substance, near the ligamentum latum, was a tumour containing a tea spoonful of very thin, subalbid fluid; the sides of the cavity were of a pale grey colour, and much softened, to the extent of half an inch. The colon, thickened, contracted, and covered with numerous large grey ulcers. (*Twining, Diseases of Bengal*, vol. i, *p*. 311.)

No. 290.—M. Victor Jacquemont, the French traveller and philosopher. His case is principally interesting as showing that strictly abstemious habits, are *alone* no protection to the supervention of hepatic abscess. No one could have been more temperate; for a long time he had left off the use of spirituous liquors, discarded animal food, and lived on nearly the same diet as the natives, only in smaller quantities. He took regular walking or riding exercise, morning and evening; but living, as he was obliged to do, principally in tents, he was exposed, particularly in the hot season, to extreme heat, and to great atmospherical changes. He was first attacked with dysentery, and irregular attacks of fever; hepatic abscess supervened, and he died at Bombay, Dec. 7th, 1832, 15 hours after the rupture of the abscess into the cavity of the peritoneum. No Autopsy. (*Twining*, ibid, *p*. 326.)

No. 291.—J. McCan, æt. 20, by trade a painter, just from England, of middle stature, light complexion, delicate; admitted May 30th, 1829, with disease of the knee joint, of five months duration. Under the use of mercurial plasters to the knee, Plummer's pill at night, and purgatives, he much improved, but he remained pale and weak. July 7th, he complained of cough and shortness of breath, with scanty viscid sputa; there was no pain on pressure over the abdomen, except over the spleen; no pyrexia; tongue clean and moist; pulse 120, soft; urine scanty and high coloured, coagulating slightly when heated. Under palliative treatment he seemed to improve up to Aug. 8th, when profuse purging came on, followed by some heat of skin, pain in the temples, and morbid sensibility on pressure over the cæcum—abdomen full, not elastic but *doughy*—tongue moist, and slightly fissured. The report on Aug. 11th, is "pulse 90, belly slightly retracted, has pain in the right shoulder and down the arm, which was first felt the day before;"—20th, a slight hardness of the liver observed, the right rectus muscle more tense than the left; he was pale, emaciated and weak;—24th, had a rigor, (for the first time,) vomited frequently, and had six stools with a slight appearance of pus in them; pulse from 120 to 126;—27th, copious perspiration, hectic flush, tongue morbidly red;—31st, the enlargement of the right lobe more prominent;—Sept. 3d, had a troublesome cough, with copious expectoration of yellow muco-purulent matter, of "a bitter stinking taste;" the tumour of the liver less prominent, and he felt easier; urine of a deep colour, with a white powdery sediment;—on the 5th, the cough had decreased, and he expectorated a thin oily matter, slightly tinged with greenish yellow bile. Died Sept. 7th, 1829.

Autopsy.—Liver enlarged, adherent to the diaphragm, through which an abscess had opened into the right lung; this was much decreased in size, and contained many suppurating tubercles; the left lung also contained tubercles. Gall-bladder elongated and flaccid, and contained some straw-coloured fluid like varnish; coats of the cæcum thickened and ulcerated. Mesenteric glands enlarged. (*Twining*, ibid, vol. i, *p.* 356.)

No. 292.—A seaman, admitted with dysentery into the General Hospital in Calcutta; died in 13 days. History of the case not given.

Autopsy.—Liver much enlarged, containing a large abscess in the right lobe—gall-bladder half full of greenish thin bile—much ulceration in the cæcum and sigmoid flexure of the colon—coats thickened and easily torn. (*Dr. Macpherson, on Bengal Dysentery*, No. 2.)

No. 293.—A pauper, æt. 31, died of dysentery of 21 days duration. No history of the case.

Autopsy.—Liver contained three abscesses, two in the left lobe and one in the right lobe. Large intestines greatly altered, in some places very thin—folds of the transverse colon ulcerated. Small intestines healthy. Meso-colon injected. (*Dr. Macpherson,* ibid, No. 61.)

No. 294.—A sailor, æt. 25, died of dysentery, of ten days duration. No history of the case.

Autopsy.—The left lobe of the liver contained a small abscess. Spleen enlarged. Large intestines ulcerated and thickened throughout, chiefly in the transverse colon. (*Dr. Macpherson,* ibid, No. 80.)

No. 295.—A sailor, æt. 26, died of dysentery, after an illness of a month. No history of the case.

Autopsy.—The surface of the liver shewed recent cicatrices; in the right lobe was an extensive abscess. The large intestines in a sloughing state throughout, (*Dr. Macpherson,* ibid, No. 88.)

No. 296.—A recruit, æt. 23, admitted with dysentery, of which he had been ill some time; died 5 days after admission. No history given.

Autopsy.—Liver a little enlarged and full of abscesses, from the size of a pea to that of a nutmeg, especially on the upper surface of the right lobe. Small intestines and stomach blanched, but on the inner coat of the latter were patches of red—cæcum much thickened and ulcerated—a few superficial ulcers in the colon. (*Dr. Macpherson,* ibid, No. 107.)

No. 297.—A pauper, ill several months with chronic dysentery, died six days after admission into hospital.

Autopsy.—In the right lobe of the liver were three abscesses, full of curdy matter; large intestines thickened and ulcerated. (*Dr. Macpherson,* ibid, *p.* 36.)

No. 298.—An invalid, several weeks in hospital, discharged, but returned with a relapse of dysentery.

Autopsy.—Abscess in the liver communicating with the ascending colon; cæcum rotten and perforated, transverse colon ulcerated; sigmoid flexure healthy. (*Dr. Macpherson,* ibid, *p.* 37.)

No. 299.—An invalid, æt. 31, many months ill with dysentery.

Autopsy.—Liver double its natural size, "like a coagulum of blood;" in its substance were nine small abscesses, containing 3 or 4 ounces of pus. Small intestines healthy; large intestines slightly ulcerated; some thickening of the cæcum. (*Dr. Macpherson*, ibid, *p*. 38.)

No. 300.—— ——, æt. 22, died of chronic dysentery of 7 weeks duration. History of the case not given.

Autopsy.—Liver enlarged—a large abscess on the lower surface of the right lobe. Coats of the large intestines thin and friable, and ulcerated throughout. Mesenteric glands enlarged. (*Dr. Macpherson*, ibid.)

ANALYSIS

OF THE PRECEDING THREE HUNDRED

FATAL CASES OF HEPATIC ABSCESS.

Sex.				
	Males	291	or 97.000	per cent.
	Females (a)	9	or 3.000	per cent.
		300	100.000	

It is worthy of note, that of the nine cases occurring in females, three are stated to have been born in India; whilst, out of 291 cases in males, only six were natives of that country.

Nation. Of 57 cases in which the nation of the patient is mentioned, there were

Englishmen	20	or 35.087	per cent.
Irishmen	24	or 42.107	,,
Scotchmen	1	or 1.754	,,
Portuguese and French	3	or 5.263	,,
Indian born (b)	9	or 15.789	,,
	57	100	

Of the nine patients, Indian born, six appear to have been pure natives, either Hindoos or Mussulmen. (66, 214, 234, 256, 286, 287.) The others were Indo-Britons, or persons born in India of European parents.

It will be seen that only one Scotchman (No. 168) appears in the above list; this is partly to be accounted for by the comparatively small number of Scotchmen borne upon the strength of our regiments in India, and partly by their greater hardihood of constitution, and their more abstemious habits. Many names, undoubtedly Scotch, appear in the cases, as Kennedy, (44,) Hamilton, (71,) Campbell, (100,) and Macdonald, (165, 251,) but as the nations of these men are not specified, this particular has been omitted by me altogether.

(a) Females, cases 105, 126, 173, 178, 180, 182, 244, 254, 287.
(b) Indian-born, cases 66, 91, 178, 180, 214, 234, 256, 286, 287.

The ages of the patients at the period of death are specified in 227 cases. The following are the results :—

From 16 to 20 years of age	10	or	4.405	per cent.
,, 21 to 25 ,, ,, ...	59	or	25.000	,,
,, 26 to 30 ,, ,, ...	53	or	23.392	,,
,, 31 to 35 ,, ,, ...	42	or	18.502	,,
,, 36 to 40 ,, ,, ...	35	or	15.860	,,
,, 41 to 45 ,, ,, ...	13	or	5.727	,,
,, 46 to 50 ,, ,, ...	9	or	3.964	,,
,, 51 to 55 ,, ,, ...	2	or	0.881	,,
,, 56 to 70 ,, ,, ...	3	or	1.321	,,
72 years of age	1	or	0.440	,,
	227		100.000	

The youngest ages at which I have found any record of abscess in the liver are 16 years (Case 244) and 17 years (Case 128) respectively. Childhood may be regarded as almost, if not entirely, exempt from the invasion of suppurative inflammation of the liver. The greatest age in the above record is 72 years. (Case 101.). After the age of 50, it is rare to meet with hepatic abscess, excepting in those who lead irregular or intemperate lives. It will be observed that nearly one-half (112 out of 227) of the deaths from this cause, took place in the ten years between 20 and 30. After the latter age the number of deaths gradually decreases.

The age on arrival in India is mentioned in 100 cases; and, taken in connexion with the preceding table, it may prove interesting—by itself, it presents us with no fact of any importance.

Under 16 years	2
From 16 to 18 years	6
,, 18 to 20 ,, ...	20
,, 20 to 22 ,, ...	14
,, 22 to 24 ,, ...	17
,, 24 to 26 ,, ...	13
,, 26 to 28 ,, ...	12
,, 28 to 30 ,, ...	6
,, 30 to 35 ,, ...	6
,, 35 to 40 ,, ...	2
,, 40 to 45 ,, ...	1
,, 45 to 50 ,, ...	1
	100

From this it appears, that those who arrive in India between 18 and 24 years of age, are the most liable to hepatic abscess—but we must not overlook the fact, that it is at about this age, that by far the greater number of recruits are sent to India; and in the absence of the strength of each class, no deduction can be fairly drawn.

The length of service or residence in India is mentioned in 114 cases; of these there were

Under 1 year	26	or	22.807	per cent.
From 1 to 2 years	12	or	10.526	,,
,, 2 to 3 ,, ...	12	or	10.526	,,
,, 3 to 4 ,, ...	6	or	5.263	,,
,, 4 to 5 ,, ...	6	or	5.263	,,
,, 5 to 6 ,, ...	5	or	4.387	,,
,, 6 to 7 ,, ...	7	or	6.140	,,
,, 7 to 8 ,, ...	5	or	4.387	,,
,, 8 to 9 ,, ...	8	or	7.017	,,
,, 9 to 10 ,, ...	2	or	1.754	,,
,, 10 to 15 ,, ...	13	or	11.403	,,
,, 15 to 20 ,, ...	7	or	6.140	,,
25 years	3 }			
27 years	1 }	or	4.387	,,
28 years	1 }			
	114		100.000	

From this it appears that by far the larger proportion of cases of hepatic abscess occurs in those, whose period of service in India is very limited. Of the above number, nearly 23 per cent. died under one years residence, and more than 50 per cent. within the first four years. A larger number died in the first year, than during the ten years between 10 and 20. Length of residence in India seems to confer a great immunity from suppuration of the liver; and, when it does occur in those who have been long in India, it is almost invariably associated with irregular and intemperate habits. This is mentioned as having been the case with the man who had been resident 28 years, (No. 228,) and also in one who was of 25 years service, (No. 225.) The habits of the remaining three cases, occurring after 20 years service, are not specified.

The temperament or habit of body is mentioned in 70 cases; of these there were

Robust, large made, muscular, corpulent, ruddy, healthy, stout, or full habit ...	32	or 45.714 per cent.
Slender, slight, weak, feeble habit, sickly, delicate, and spare	25	or 35.714 per cent.
Scrofulous or strumous	3	or 18.572 per cent. (Scrofulous to Broken down)
Sanguine	3	
Melancholic	2	
Bilious	1	
Leucophlegmatic	2	
Broken down	2	
	70	100.000

With respect to complexion, there were

Fair skins, light hair, blue eyes, &c., ...	11
Swarthy, dark, or sallow, ...	8
	19

On this subject, as confirmatory of the above limited data, a short passage from Dr. Nicholls' Essay on Hepatitis* may not be out of place. "In the 80th Regt.," he observes, "those of a florid complexion, scrofulous habit, and the tall and melancholy, have suffered most from disease of the liver. During our stay at Quilon, the Grenadiers (average height 5 feet 10 inches) lost more men from abscess in the liver, in proportion to their number, than any other nine companies of the Regt. In the years 1814 and 1816, ten "good looking grenadiers," as they were called, died of abscess of the liver."

The habits and character, are specified in 40 cases. Of this limited number, there were

Temperate, sober, steady, and well conducted, ..	13	or 32.5 per cent.
Intemperate	20	27 or 67.5 per cent. (Intemperate to Dissipated)
Irregular	2	
Rather intemperate	1	
Dissipated..	4	
	40	100.00

These data are too limited to allow us to found any opinion on them; but they tend to support, in a very strong manner, the supposition that intemperance is a very fruitful source of hepatic affections in India.

At the same time, it is a well ascertained fact, that temperate

* Madras Quarterly Medical Journal, vol. iii, p. 256.

habits, and a regular, steady, and sober life, by no means confer exemption from the invasion of suppurative inflammation of the liver. Of this we have examples in cases 18, 19, 131, 132, &c., but none illustrates this point so forcibly as case 290.

The influence of previous occupation, whether in-door or out-door, is not very marked. Taking the cases of 45, (most of them soldiers,) we find that their occupations in Europe were

In-door. .	Weavers, 3; Tailors, 2; Flaxdresser, 1; Ironsmiths, 2; Schoolmaster, 1; Plumber, 1; Clothdresser, 1; Clerks, 3; Cotton-spinner, 1; Silk-dyer, 1; Shoemaker, 1; Painter, 1	18
Out-door	Labourers, 14; Bricklayer, 1; Farrier, 1; Butcher, 1	17
	Musician, 1; Servants, 2 ... ... Gentlemen, 5; Surgeons, 2	10
		45

In addition to these, there died of hepatic abscess in the General Hospitals of Calcutta, Madras, and Bombay, no fewer than 34 sailors, men proverbial for their irregular lives, and who are, of necessity, exposed to great vicissitudes of climate and temperature, and that too, generally under the most unfavourable circumstances.

Of the average duration of these cases, we have the means of judging in 220 cases; partly from the length of time that they were actually under treatment, and partly from the previous history of the case, as given by the patient himself. In some cases, in consequence of the obscurity of the symptoms, and the insidious character of the disease, we have had to judge entirely from the length of time that the patient remained in hospital: this was the case with all those patients who were a very short time in hospital.

Under 5 days	4
From 5 to 10 days	25
,, 10 to 20 ,, ...	59
,, 20 to 30 ,, ...	37
,, 30 to 40 ,, ...	29
,, 40 to 50 ,, ...	12
,, 50 to 60 ,, ...	14
,, 60 to 70 ,, ...	10
,, 70 to 80 ,, ...	5
,, 80 to 100 ,, ...	11
,, 100 to 120 ,, ...	9
Above 120 days	5
	220

The total number of days that these 220 cases were under treatment, was 8196; giving an average of between 38 and 39 days to each case.

The shortest period of stay in hospital was 5¼ hours; (No. 66) in fact, the man was moribund at the time of admission. After death, there was found in his liver an immense abscess, containing two pints of matter. We shall have occasion to refer to this case, when considering the insidious and obscure characters of the symptoms.

In the very lengthy cases, particularly in those above 120 days, (Cases 68, 212, 227, 229,) the symptoms were generally of a very varying and anomalous character. The longest period of stay in hospital was 192 days. (Case 212.)

Months of Admission and Death. The months in which 216 cases of fatal hepatic abscess were admitted.

Cold Months.		*Hot Months.*		*Rainy Months.*	
November ...	19	March ...	13	July ...	21
December ...	30	April ...	18	August ...	21
January ...	23	May ...	18	September ...	19
February ...	9	June ...	9	October ...	16
	81		58		77
Per cent...	37.50	Per cent...	26.85	Per cent...	35.65

Months of death in 243 cases.

Cold Months.		*Hot Months.*		*Rainy Months.*	
November ...	34	March ...	11	July ...	16
December ...	17	April ...	14	August ...	19
January ...	32	May ...	18	September ...	20
February ...	18	June ...	20	October ...	24
	101		63		79
Per cent...	41.56	Per cent...	25.92	Per cent...	32.51

From this it appears that the maximum, both of deaths and admissions, is in the cold months; and the minimum, in both cases is in the hot months.

The diseases which immediately preceded the formation of abscess in the liver, or during the progress of which hepatic suppuration supervened, are as follows :—

	No.	Per cent.
Hepatitis, Acute and Chronic	131	or 43.666
Dysentery, Acute and Chronic	82	or 27.333
Dysentery and Hepatitis, or Hepatic Dysentery	14	or 4.666
Fever, or Common Continued Fever	14	or 4.666
Intermittent Fever	5	or 1.666
Remittent Fever	3	or 1.000
Diarrhœa or Purging	6	or 2.333 (with next)
Diarrhœa and Intermittent Fever	1	
Admitted with Hepatic Abscess evidently formed	6	or 2.000
Catarrh and Catarrhal Fever	2	or 6.333 (with following, to Pneumonia)
Delirium Tremens	2	
Rheumatism	2	
Abdominal Inflammation	2	
Constipation	2	
Constipation and a swelling simulating Ventral Hernia	1	
Injury of the side from contusion or fall	3	
Ulcer on the leg followed by Dysentery	1	
Disease of the Brain	1	
Acute Ophthalmia	1	
Disease of the knee joint	1	
Pneumonia (?) following unusual exertion	1	
Doubtful	19	or 6.333
	300	100.000

From this Table it is evident that the proportion of cases of hepatic abscess occuring after or during the progress of hepatitis, dysentery, and fever is not only much larger than that of any other disease, but of all diseases put together; I believe this to be also in accordance with the experience and observation of medical men in India generally.

It ought perhaps to be stated, that in enumerating the cases of admission with hepatitis, some latitude has been used by me, as in the histories of some of the cases from which this Table is compiled, it is not on the face of them, expressly stated that the patient was admitted with hepatitis; but, simply, that the patient was admitted with severe or acute pain in the right hypochondrium, increased or not by pressure or full inspiration, hot skin, &c., of so many days standing—such cases as these I have assumed to be hepatitis. Those about which any doubt could be reasonably entertained, have been classed as doubtful.

The following interesting Table framed by the late Dr. J. Mouat, (see *Madras Medical Journal,* volume ii, page 9,) strongly corroborates the results given above.

Return of Casualties in H. M. 13th Dragoons, from January 1826 to December 1838—noting the condition of the liver in each case.

Diseases.	Total deaths from each disease.	State of liver on post-mortem examination. Abscess.	Structural disease.*	Healthy.	No dissection report.
Febris Remittens Biliosa ..	22	2	14	6	0
„ Continua Communis.	3	0	1	2	0
„ Typhus	1	0	0	0	1
Phrenitis	1	0	1	0	0
Pneumonia	7	0	4	2	1
Gastritis..............	6	0	5	0	1
Enteritis..............	2	0	0	2	0
Hepatitis Acuta.........	58	51	5	0	2
„ Chronica	2	0	0	0	2
Rheumatismus Acutus....	1	0	0	0	1
Hæmoptysis	2	1	1	0	0
Phthisis Pulmonalis......	8	0	5	3	0
Dysenteria Acuta........	67	13	30	18	6
Apoplexia..............	5	0	3	2	0
Paralysis...............	5	0	3	1	1
Epilepsia..............	1	0	1	0	0
Asthma Periodica........	1	0	1	0	0
Cholera Communis.......	2	0	2	0	0
„ Pestilentia.......	47	0	13	26	8
Diarrhœa	7	1	3	0	3
Anasarca	4	0	4	0	0
Ascites	1	0	0	0	1
Syphilis Consecutiva.....	1	0	0	1	0
Aneurisma Aortæ.........	4	0	3	1	0
Vulnus Incisum..........	1	0	0	1	0
Concussio Cerebri........	4	0	2	2	0
Compressio Cerebri......	1	0	1	0	0
Delirium Tremens.......	4	0	3	1	0
	268	68	105	68	27

* Namely enlargement, induration, softening, congestion, discolorations, adhesions, granulations, &c.

From the two preceding Tables we are justified in regarding hepatitis as the disease which, in the most marked manner, originates abscess in the liver; or, in other words, during the progress of which, hepatic abscess supervenes;—thus, out of 300 collected histories, the abscess commenced in connexion with hepatitis in 131 instances, or in nearly 44 per cent—and, on the other hand, we see from the second Table, that in 56 cases of fatal hepatitis, in which the body was examined, abscess was present in 51 cases, or in above 91 per cent. I regret that I have no further statistical evidence, at present, to substantiate the point; but I imagine that the foregoing data are sufficiently strong, to prove, beyond a reasonable doubt, the extreme frequency of abscess in the liver as a sequence of hepatitis. This is a result that might, *a priori*, have been anticipated. Good examples of the mode in which this occurs, and the symptoms attendant on the formation of abscess in these cases, are to be found in Nos. 12, 41, 58, 97.

With respect to the connexion between hepatic abscess and dysentery, our information is more extensive. We shall subsequently see that, out of a certain number of hepatic abscesses, ulceration of the large intestines, the most constant of all pathological appearances in tropical dysentery, was present in 72 per cent; but in many of these cases there appears little doubt that the bowel affection supervened upon the hepatic; (as in cases 15, 19, 54, 91, 163, 209,) and our present enquiry is rather to ascertain the number of cases in which dysentery was the primary affection. The following Table tends to throw much light on the subject :—

Table showing the Proportion of cases of fatal Dysentery in Madras, Bengal, and Bombay, in which abscess of the Liver was found on Post-mortem examination.

Presidency	Station.	Regiment or Hospital.	Date.	No. of fatal cases of Dysentery.	No. in which abscess in the liver was found.	Proportion.	Proportion in each Presidency.	Authority.
Madras.	Secunderabad.	H. M. 55th Regt.	1837	96	36	1 in $3\frac{7}{10}$		Dr. Shanks, Mad. Med. Journal, i, 258.
	Ditto.	H. M. 4th Regt.	1843	43	8	1 in $5\frac{3}{10}$		Dr. Innis, Do. do. do. vi, 172.
	Bangalore, &c.	H. M. 13th Drags.	1826–38	61	13	1 in $4\frac{3}{5}$		Dr. Mouat, Do. do. do. ii, 9.
	Cannanore.	H. M. 54th Regt.	1828	17	0	,,		Dr. Hamilton, Do. do. do. iv, 318.
	Ditto.	H. M. 94th Regt.	1840	26	9	1 in $2\frac{9}{10}$		Mr. Dix, Do. do. do. v, 214.
	Trichinopoly.	H. M. 54th Regt.	1834	11	2	1 in $5\frac{1}{2}$		Mr. Thompson Do. do. do. v, 16.
	Bangalore.	H. M. 39th Regt.	1836	5	1	1 in 5	Madras	Mr. McGregor Do. do. do. ii, 376.
				259	69	....	1 in 3.754	
Bengal.	Calcutta.	Seaman's Hospl.	....	24	5	1 in $4\frac{2}{3}$		Dr. Macpherson, On Dysentery, 49.
	Ditto.	Med. Coll. Hospl.	....	54	14	1 in $3\frac{4}{5}$		Dr. Macpherson, Do. do.
	Ditto.	General Hospital.	....	215	27	1 in 8	Bengal	Dr. Macpherson, Do. do.
				293	46	....	1 in 6.369	[Phys. Soc. vii, 56.
Bombay.	Bombay.	Eur. Gen. Hospl.	1840–43	32	13	1 in $2\frac{2}{5}$		Dr. Morehead, Trans. of Bom. Med. &
	Ditto.	Ditto.	1847	10	3	1 in $3\frac{3}{10}$		Dr. Stovell, Do. ix, 49.
	Ditto.	Ditto.	1850–51	15	5	1 in 3		Dr. Stovell, Do. No. 1, N.S. 297.
	Ditto.	Ditto.	1851–52	24	13	1 in $1\frac{9}{10}$	Bombay	Dr. Stovell, Do. do.
				81	34	....	1 in 2.382	
						General Average		
	Total.	....	....	633	149	1 in 4.241		

This Table presents several points for consideration. First, it would appear that the complication of hepatic abscess with dysentery, is most frequent in Bombay, and least so in Calcutta; whilst Madras holds an intermediate place. Secondly, in two hospitals in the same station or locality, *e. g.* the Medical College Hospital and the General Hospital, both in Calcutta, a great discrepancy exists as to the frequency of this complication; being in the former establishment under 4 per cent, and in the latter 8 per cent—and, Thirdly, in two successive years, in the same hospital, the Bombay European General Hospital, 1850—51 and 52, and it is to be presumed, amongst the same class of patients, there exists a wide difference as to the frequency of this complication. Can the mode of treatment adopted be sufficient to account for these discrepancies?

Some further, but brief observations on this interesting subject may be acceptable.

In the first Burmese war, 1824-25, Dr. G. Waddell,(a) states that he did not find disease of the liver in any one of his dissections of those who died of the dysentery which proved so fatal to our troops. In the last Burmese war, 1852-53, Mr. Stewart, (b) of H. M. 18th Royal Irish, states that in fully three-fourths of the fatal cases of dysentery, the liver was found more or less implicated, from simple engorgement to abscess. The latter statement is borne out by Dr. Taylor, (c) of H. M. 80th Regiment. Of 24 cases of fatal dysentery examined by this gentleman, 4 presented abscess of the liver.

Of 61 fatal cases of dysentery, dissected by Dr. John Wilson,(d) in China, hepatic abscess was found in two instances only.

In the epidemic dysentery which prevailed in Dublin, in 1818, Dr. Cheyne (e) met with hepatic abscess in 4 cases, out of 30 bodies examined.

Out of many hundred cases of dysentery examined by Dr. Baly,(f) which occurred in the Milbank Penitentiary during seven years, (1840-47,) not one was complicated with hepatic abscess.

Of 64 cases of chronic dysentery, from India, Ceylon, and the Coast of Africa, examined by Dr. Knox,(g) of Edinburgh, the liver was diseased in two only.

(a) Trans. of Med. and Phys. Society of Calcutta, vol. iii, p. 254.
(b) Indian Annals of Med. Science, 1854, No. 2, p. 434.
(c) Ibid, No. 2, p. 394.
(d) Medical Notes on China, London, 1846, p. 258.
(e) Dublin Hospital Reports, vol. iii.
(f) Gulstonian Lectures, Medical Gazette, vol. iv, p. 485.
(g) Abercrombie on Diseases of the Stomach, &c., 3d Ed. p. 243.

Dr. Abercrombie, (*Diseases of the Stomach, &c. 3d Ed. p. 243*) states that of all his dissections of dysenteric patients in Great Britain, he never saw the liver affected, except in one or two chronic cases.

Rokitansky(a) also states that in all his dissections of cases of dysentery, he never found the liver visibly diseased.

In estimating the frequency of the complication now under consideration, I have purposely omitted the cases detailed by Annesley and Twining; for the simple reason, that they are *selected* cases; all that we are entitled to say, after perusing these histories, so given, is, that a certain number of abscesses in the liver were found in so many cases of fatal dysentery: we have no clue afforded us by which we may judge of the *total number of dysenteric deaths*, and until we have this, any deductions drawn from these cases must be fallacious.

The symptoms which mark the supervention of hepatic abscess in cases of dysentery, are often very obscure; it seems most frequently to occur during the period of convalescence. See cases 9, 18, 35, 39, 40, 111, 140, 167, 235, &c. In others (161, 166,) the dysenteric symptoms are so severe, that they mask the hepatic symptoms altogether.

We cannot conclude this portion of the subject without alluding to the views of Dr. Budd, on the connection between these two diseases. He considers that abscess in the liver arises from pre-existing ulceration of some part of the intestines, stomach, or gall-bladder; parts which return their blood to the portal vein, to be thence transmitted through the capillaries of the liver: that this secondary affection of the liver does not arise from the spreading of the inflammation, but from some contamination of the portal blood: that this noxious agent, may be either pus, formed by suppurative inflammation of one of the small intestinal veins; or matter of other kinds, resulting from the softening of the tissues; or fetid, gaseous, and liquid contents of the large intestines in dysentery, which must be absorbed and conveyed immediately to the liver, (*p.* 64.)

However unsatisfactory it is to dissent from a plausible explanation, when the person so dissenting has no other or better explanation to offer, yet, with respect to the above proposition, I am bound to state that it does not appear to me to unravel the mysterious tie by which these two diseases are connected.

1. If this hypothesis were correct, abscess of the liver would occur much more frequently than it does, in the course of dysen-

(*a*) Med. Jahrbücher des Oesterreich Staates, Bd. xx, 1840, p. 81.

tery. The following short Table, having reference only to the Madras Presidency, will tend to place this subject in its true light. It may be regarded as a continuation of the last Table.

Regiment.	Date.	No. of cases of Dysentery treated.	Deaths from Dysentery.	No. in which abscess in the liver was found.	Per centage of abscess in liver to No. of cases treated.	Authority.
H. M. 55th Regt.	1837	436	96	36	8.256	Dr. Shanks.
H. M. 4th Regt.	1843	224	43	8	3.587	Dr. Innis.
H. M. 13th Drags.	1826–38	1448	67	13	0.898	Dr. Mouat.
H. M. 54th Regt.	1828	294	17	0	0.000	Dr. Hamilton.
H. M. 54th Regt.	1840	148	11	2	1.351	Dr. Thompson.
H. M. 94th Regt.	1834	208	26	9	4.327	Dr. Dix.
		2758	260	68	2.462	

From this it appears that out of 2758 cases of dysentery treated in the Madras Presidency, abscess of the liver occurred 68 times, being in the proportion of 2½ per cent nearly. I think that it must be admitted that if Dr. Budd's explanation were the true one, the proportion would be very much larger than this return shows it to be, and we must therefore look for some other and more predominant cause, than the one which he has so ingeniously supplied.

2. On referring to the preceding histories, we find that out of 204 cases in which the state of the large intestines is described, they were not in a state of ulceration, being generally healthy in 51 or in about 25 per cent.

3. Looking at the diseases under which the patients were admitted in 300 instances, we find hepatitis recorded as the primary affection in 131, (or 43 per cent,) whilst only 82 (or 27 per cent,) were admissions from dysentery.

4. Although it must be admitted that in the majority of cases, some derangement of the bowels was coeval with, or even anterior to, the evident manifestation of hepatic abscess, yet in several instances, Nos. 15, 19, 54, 91 and 163, for example, the dysenteric symptoms did not appear till an advanced stage of the disease, and in some not until the existence of abscess was placed almost beyond a doubt.

At the same time that I feel it necessary, from the above facts, to dissent from Dr. Budd's views on this subject, still less am I prepared to admit Annesley's explanation, namely, that the ulceration of the bowels arises from the passage of vitiated or irritating bile, for, as Dr. Budd justly observes, if this were the case, we should expect to find the most evident marks of the disease in the gall-ducts and upper part of the small intestines, parts with which the irritating matter came first in contact; but instead of this, these parts are almost always healthy in cases in which abscess in the liver is associated with the most destructive forms of dysentery. Case No. 5 is the best refutation of this hypothesis, that I have met with; here the gall-bladder was involved in the suppurative process, had been removed by gangrene, and the abscess opened directly into the colon; the intestine was found distended with dark gangrenous fluid, and yet its mucous coat showed no sign of ulceration.

I am inclined to think that Dr. Parkes' explanation will be found eventually to approximate nearer to the truth. He suggests that there exists a reciprocity of secretive and excretive action between the liver and the colon; that the chemical constitution of the blood, in consequence of the non-action of the solitary glands of the large intestines, becomes altered, and that the blood thus chemically changed, has a tendency to produce hepatic abscess. Of course this explanation must remain in part hypothetical, till further advances have been made in animal chemistry.

Many patients appear to have been in hospital once or oftener with hepatic disease, before their admission with the fatal attack. Of 36 cases we find that:—

Seven(a)	or 19.444	per cent	had been	treated for	hepatic disease	once
Three(b)	or 8.333	per cent	,,	,,	,,	twice
Five(c)	or 13.900	per cent	,,	,,	,,	three times
Three(d)	or 8.333	per cent	,,	,,	,,	four times
One(e)	or 2.777	per cent	,,	,,	,,	five times
Two(f)	or 5.555	per cent	,,	,,	,,	six times
One(g)	or 2.777	per cent	,,	,,	,,	seven times
Two(h)	or 5.555	per cent	,,	,,	,,	eight times
One(i)	or 2.777	per cent	,,	,,	,,	thirteen times
Eleven(j)	or 30.833	per cent	,,	,,		repeatedly or often

In only three instances is it mentioned that the patient had never before been under treatment for hepatic disease, until admitted with the fatal attack. (Cases 36, 44, 215.)

From the history of many of the cases in which the patients were often in hospital with hepatic disease, (especially cases 48 and 262) it may reasonably be inferred that abscess in the liver may remain

(a) Cases 19, 27, 30, 64, 184, 202, 204. (b) Cases 6, 23, 209.
(c) Cases 50, 173, 194, 190, 228. (d) Cases 21, 192, 229.
(e) Case 208. (f) Cases 187, 196. (g) Case 201.
(h) Cases 191, 203. (i) Case 189. (j) Cases 25, 42, 87, 96, 103, 177, 225, 230, 262.

stationary for years, and that it is only after the application of some powerfully existing cause, that it assumes an active character, and progresses to its termination.

Abscess in the liver is not confined to the human species. In the museum of the Calcutta Medical College, the preparations in which form the ground work of Dr. Allan Webb's Pathologia Indica, are several specimens of the liver of the common rat, affected with abscess. The liver of a dog, containing tubercles of a pulpy or scrofulous character, is also preserved; and likewise the liver of an orang-outang, in which suppuration had disorganized one of the many lobes of that viscus. In this last case the abscess communicated with the right kidney. (*See Path. Indica, p.* 257, *et seq.*)

The number of abscesses found in each case.

	No.	Per cent.	
One, single or solitary ...	177	59.000	per cent.
Two abscesses	33	11.000	,,
Three ,, ...	11	3.666	,,
Four ,, ...	17	5.666	,,
Five ,, ...	5	1.666	,,
Six ,, ...	1	0.333	,,
Seven ,, ...	1	0.333	,,
Eight ,, ...	1	0.333	,,
Nine ,, ...	1	0.333	,,
Ten ,, ...	1	0.333	,,
Eighteen ,, ...	1	0.333	,,
Numerous ,, ...	36	12.000	,,
Diffused ,, ...	3	1.000	,,
Number not stated, or doubtful	12	4.000	,,
	300	100.000	,,

This Table is of great importance in a practical point of view, especially with reference to the advisability of performing the operation for the purpose of evacuating the contents of an abscess. We see from it that:—

A single abscess existed in 177 cases, or in 62.105 per cent.
Numerous abscesses in 108 cases, or in 37.895 per cent.

In estimating this last per centage, the fifteen cases included under the last two headings have been omitted; it would have been obviously incorrect to have admitted these into the calculation, when considering simply the relative frequency of single and numerous abscesses.

The position of these abscesses in the liver with reference to the lobes, was as follows :—

Right lobe	...163	or	67.355	per cent.
Left lobe	... 16	or	6.611	,,
Right and left lobes ...	... 35	or	14.462	,,
Between the right and left lobes, under the ligamentum latum	... 4	or	1.652	,,
Right and middle lobes ...	... 1	or	0.414	,,
Left and middle lobes ...	... 1	or	0.414	,,
Right, left, and middle lobes	... 1	or	0.414	,,
Lobulus Spigelii ...	... 1	or	0.414	,,
Abscesses throughout the liver	... 20	or	8.264	,,
Diffused abscesses ...	... 3	omitted.		
Exact site not given ...	... 50			
No post-mortem ...	... 5			
	300			

From this it appears that of 242 cases, 67 per cent of these abscesses existed in the right lobe of the liver alone ; but, if we take into consideration the large number of other cases in which this lobe, conjointly with some other portion of the liver, was the seat of abscess, the proportion is indeed enormous. At the same time we should bear in mind, the great relative size of the right lobe to the other lobes of the liver.

The frequency of abscess in this lobe is no new fact; it was observed above half a century ago by Sir James McGrigor, in his account of the diseases of the 88th Regt. &c. (Annals of Medicine for 1801, *p.* 363,) and the fact was further illustrated by Dr. Geddes, in his paper on hepatic abscess, in the 6th volume of the Transactions of the Medical and Physical Society of Calcutta.

The position of the abscesses may be further considered with reference to the surfaces, borders, &c. of the liver. Thus we find that they existed :—

On the upper and superior part of the right lobe ...	in 19
On the upper and outer part of the right lobe ...	in 7
On the convex surface of the right lobe	in 11
On the concave surface of the right lobe	in 4
On the inferior edge or margin of the right lobe ...	in 4
Deep seated, or in the centre of the right lobe ...	in 2
In the upper part of the left lobe...	in 1
In the centre of the left lobe	in 1
Between the right and left lobes	in 4
On both surfaces	in 3

The general term "liver," is employed by some of the writers from whose works the above cases are extracted, and we find it stated that the abscess existed—

In the upper and posterior portion of the liver	...	in 6
In the concave surface of the liver	... ...	in 4
In the centre, or deep seated	... ...	in 2
In the centre, involving the lobulus Spigelii	...	in 1
In the convex surface of the liver	... ...	in 4

When several abscesses exist in the liver at the same time, they may occupy very various positions in that viscus. Of this numerous examples are to be found in the preceding histories, Nos. 2, 3, 117, 170, &c.

The characters of the matter found in these hepatic abscesses are so various, and the expressions employed by the different writers so multiplied, that at first it seemed almost a hopeless task to form any arrangement of them. I have, however, classed them as below, making, in a few instances, a slight change in the form of expression. Whenever the least ambiguity existed, the original expression has been allowed to remain. In 127 cases, we find the following descriptions:—

Pus, purulent matter, well digested, good, pure, healthy, white, and laudable pus, ...	48
Thick, creamy, or white, thick pus, ...	18
Sero-purulent matter, ...	6
Curdled matter, curdy, curdiform or whey-like, ...	6
Thin, flaky, purulent matter or fluid, ...	5
Dark pus, dark chocolate-like matter, dark serous,... ...	6
Coffee-like, with flakes of pus,...	4
Thick yellow, and thick yellow greenish matter, ...	6
Greenish, purulent, and brownish or reddish matter, ...	6
Fluid, like wine lees, with flakes of pus; dark yellow, very offensive; matter, mixed with sloughy shreds; turbid serous fluid; dirty, fetid pus; glutinous, dark brown, thick fluid; partly greenish, partly liverish-coloured matter; matter of various hues; reddish brown, fetid; yellow, curdly water; thick, sanious; reddish puriform; partly serous, partly puriform; lardaceous, subalbid, and cheesy matter; one each, respectively,	16
	119

In five other cases (a) hæmorrhage had taken place within the sac of the abscess, and after death the blood was found in this

(a) Cases 47, 138, 148, 226, 258.

situation; in three instances in the form of coagula, and in the remaining two it is described as "grumous blood." In two of these cases, (226, 258,) the hæmorrhage into the sac appeared to be the immediate cause of death. In the latter, the vessel through which the hæmorrhage took place, was distinctly visible on the floor of the abscess.

Bile, more or less intimately incorporated with the contents of the abscess, was found in five instances.(a)

When numerous abscesses exist in the same liver, matter of very different characters is not unfrequently found in each; we have several examples of this.(b)

Those conditions or states which may be regarded as hepatic abscess in its earliest stages, may be seen in cases 88, 90, 91, 95, and 289.

The quantity of matter contained in the abscesses is mentioned in 69 cases, and may be classed as follows; premising that 16 ounces has been considered as constituting a pint, and a pound, respectively. Thus we find

4 ounces, and under	in	6 cases.
From 4 to 8 ounces	in	4 ,,
,, 8 to 12 ,,	in	4 ,,
,, 12 to 16 ,,	in	8 ,,
,, 1 to 2 pints or pounds		16 ,,
,, 2 to 3 ,,	,,	12 ,,
,, 3 to 4 ,,	,,	5 ,,
,, 4 to 5 ,,	,,	2 ,,
,, 5 to 6 ,,	,,	6 ,,
,, 6 to 7 ,,	,,	2 ,,
A gallon (No. 59, 147)		2 ,,
A gallon and a quarter (No. 2)		1 ,,
Several pints		1 ,,
		69

Large as are the quantities in some of these cases, they are all exceeded in an instance mentioned by Mr. Inman, of Liverpool, in which the contents of the abscess amounted to thirteen pints. (*Edin. Med. and Surg. Journal*, No. clx, *p.* 140.)

The size of many of these abscesses is necessarily very large; in some, the right lobe is stated to have been converted into the sac of an enormous abscess; (No. 25, 174,) in one the sac is said to have been large enough to contain a head; (No. 235,) in others to have been the size of an ostrich's egg; (No. 91, 93, 104,) and in

(a) Cases 49, 152, 222, 233, 246. (b) Cases 45, 146, 213, 220, 233, 234, 242, &c.

others to have been 6, 7, or 8 inches in diameter; (No. 7.) It is unnecessary to produce any other examples: it is not difficult to picture the size of a sac which is capable of holding a gallon and a quarter of fluid!

The question of an abscess in the liver being encysted or unencysted, has always been regarded as a point of great importance; and it is, therefore, not a little wonderful to find the subject so often passed over in silence; or only mentioned in so vague a manner, as to leave great doubt in the mind of the reader, whether the abscess was enclosed in a cyst or not: for example, "sac of the abscess," is a term frequently met with; in some, it is evidently intended only to mean the parietes of the abscess, without any reference to the condition or character of the abscess-walls. Of 53 cases, however, in which we are able to judge—

The contents of the abscess were enclosed in a cyst in	...	36
,, ,, unencysted in	...	17
		53

The following are the descriptions given of the abscess-walls in encysted cases:—Simply encysted, or having cysts, in 7; with thickened walls, in 4; with firm membrane, or walls, in 4; with thin membranous walls, in 2; in 2, the walls were composed of organized or coagulable lymph; in 1, of albuminous or fibrinous concretions; and in 1, they were dense and fibrous. They were more or less cartilaginous and firm, in 3; cartilaginous, with flocculi adherent to the inner surface, in 2; composed of a layer of thick, curdy matter, in 1; lined with a false membrane of honey-comb structure, of a greyish colour, in 1; and in another, the lining membrane was yellow, thick, and tough, like chamois leather.

In three cases there were numerous abscesses throughout the liver, each in a separate sac or cyst. (Cases 80, 218, 240.) When two or more abscesses occur in the same liver, the cysts may be of two or more different descriptions; of this we have an example in No. 233.

Of the unencysted abscesses, the walls are described as more or less flocculent in 7; composed of dense cellular tissue in 2; of the excavated substance of the liver which was soft and dark in 1; and in another the walls were flocculent, with numerous little bloody points, which proved to be the extremities of eroded arteries. (Case 226.) In 3, the matter was diffused through the parenchyma of the liver; and in 1, it is simply stated that the abscess was without a cyst. In No. 287, there were numerous abscesses in the liver, all non-encysted.

There is a third class of cases in which it is doubtful whether the abscesses were originally encysted or not; these cases are far from uninteresting. In one case, (No. 5,) the walls were dark, livid, and gangrenous; in three others, (No. 128, 137, 244,) they were in a sloughing state; and in another, (142,) the walls were ulcerated, tearing on the slightest pressure. In one (223,) "the sac" (?) was uneven and pierced with foramina, which proved to be branches of the hepatic vein; and in another, (50,) the walls are said to have been broken down, and covered with dirty fetid pus.

With respect to the flocculent walls, above mentioned, some difference of opinion seems to exist. Dr. Morehead considers, (*Trans. of Med. and Phys. Society of Bombay*, vol. vii, *p.* 38,) that it is probably the broken down secretory substances which constitutes the flocculent shreds, so commonly found adherent to the walls of abscesses in the liver. On the other hand, Dr. Conwell, (*On the Liver, p.* 518,) regards these as the eroded extremities of small arteries; and he proved his position in part by tracing distinctly their tubular form, and by finding their calibre filled with blood, pus, &c. See on this subject, Cases 88, 89, 95, 108, 216, and 219.

The Terminations of these abscesses are as follow :—

	No.	Per Cent.
Remained intact	169	56.335
Evacuated by operation, a solitary abscess being present.	29	16.000
,, ,, there being numerous abscesses, one opened, and the others remaining intact	18	
One abscess opened by operation, another subsequently bursting into the abdominal cavity (No. 27)	1	
Opened spontaneously into the thoracic cavity	14	4.666
,, ,, into the right lung	28	9.333
,, ,, into the abdominal cavity	15	5.000
,, ,, into the colon or large intestines	7	2.333
,, ,, into the stomach (No. 243)	1	6.333
,, ,, into the hepatic vein leading to the vena cava (No. 222, 223)	2	
,, ,, into the hepatic vein at its junction with the vena cava, and another communicating with the cellular tissue around the right kidney (No. 233)	1	
Communicated with the hepatic ducts (No. 284)	1	
,, with the right kidney (No. 32, 253)	2	
,, with the gall-bladder (No. 160)	1	
,, with an abscess in the iliac region (No. 81)	1	
Opened spontaneously through the ribs in the back (No. 244)	1	
One abscess had opened into the colon, and another had passed off by the hepatic ducts into the duodenum (No. 149)	1	
One abscess had opened into the stomach, a second into the duodenum, and a third had been evacuated by operation (No. 241)	1	
One abscess had opened into the abdominal cavity, and a second into the lungs (No. 48)	1	
Terminated in erysipelas of the lower extremities, simulating phlegmasia dolens, the abscess opening into the lungs (No. 274)	1	
Doubtful	5	
	300	100.000

There are some points connected with the termination of these cases, which merit consideration. We will instance a few of the most important and interesting.

In case 148, the abscess burst into the abdominal cavity, ascites having previously supervened; the accumulated fluid was drawn off by operation, and, together with the ordinary serous fluid, the matter which had escaped from the abscess was evacuated. The operation was repeated three times, and on each occasion a similar evacuation of pus took place. After the last operation, the orifice did not heal, and from this opening, purulent matter, (evidently from the abscess in the liver,) continued to be discharged up to the period of the patient's death, 19 days after the first evacuation of purulent matter.

In case 35, a small abscess in the liver had given way, and the matter escaped between the parietes of the abdomen and the intestines, until it had reached the inside of the rim of the pelvis, where its further progress was arrested; the inflammation which immediately took place confined it in this position, so that after death, when the body was examined, from 4 to 6 ounces of pus were found, extending in a direct line of about four inches in breadth, from the opening in the liver to about Poupart's ligament. The man survived the bursting of the abscess about 16 days.

In cases 47, 226 and 258, the immediate cause of death appears to have been hæmorrhage into the sac of the abscess. No. 47 is peculiarly interesting; for some days previous to death, the patient had passed blood both in his stools and also by vomiting;—on dissection, on the most minute search, no point could be found either in the intestines or stomach, from which the blood passed by stool and retching, could have oozed; the stomach and small intestines were perfectly healthy, but on the mucous coat of the duodenum were observed some small clots of blood—its structure however was unchanged in any way. The gall-bladder was also healthy, but was distended and contained coagula of blood—these were likewise found in the sac of the abscess;—it appears certain that the hæmorrhage must first have taken place into the sac of the abscess—that the blood must have passed by the biliary vessels into the gall-bladder, and thence by the ductus communis into the duodenum.

In case 173, a small tumour appeared in the right dorsal region, over the angles of the 7th and 8th ribs—this was opened, and there was a considerable discharge of pus, evidently traceable to the abscess in the liver.

Case 240 is peculiarly interesting, the patient dying from an abscess in the brain, which evidently supervened upon an abscess in the liver.

Case 274 is important in many respects—terminating as it did in phlebitis, in erysipelas of the foot, and gangrene. After death, the veins of the limb were found thickened and inflamed from the foot to the groin, and filled with coagula—the abscess had also burst into the lungs.

It may not be out of place to mention here case 288, in which the patient became extremely debilitated, and in an endeavour to turn himself in bed, *fractured his femur in an oblique direction*—union could not be established, and after death, the bone was found to be in a state of caries, and so soft that parts of it could be rubbed to powder between the thumb and finger.

Other terminations than those enumerated above, are recorded by various authors.

Cases in which the abscess opened into the pericardium, are recorded by the late Prof. Graves, of Dublin; (*Dublin Med. Journ.*, No. xiv, *p.* 349, and *Clin. Lect.*, 2d Ed., vol. ii, *p.* 233;) by Mr. Allan, Staff Surgeon, Port Louis, Mauritius; (*Lancet*, vol. i, N. S., *p.* 645;) by Dr. J. Murray, in India; (*Madras Med. Journ.*, vol. ii, *p.* 83;) by Dr. Bentley; (*Med. Gazette*, Dec. 22d, 1848, and *Ranking's Abstract*, vol. ix, *p.* 249;) by Dr. Allan Webb; (*Path. Indica*, *p.* 261;) and by Andral, (*Path. Anatomy*, translation by Townsend and West, vol. ii, *p.* 598.) In Dr. B[illegible] case, the patient appears to have survived the bursting of [illegible] abscess for thirteen hours. Dr. Webb's case is further mentioned in the List of Operations, case lxxx.

The abscess may open spontaneously through the abdominal parietes. Dr. Fuller, (*Medical Gazette*, vol. iv, N. S. *p.* 581,) relates a case in which it opened at the umbilicus; on firm pressure over the liver, large quantities of pus escaped. After death, the abscess was found in the lower margin of the liver. A very similar case, the opening being described as being near the umbilicus, is mentioned by Dr. Bristowe. (*Medical Times*, March 6th, 1852.)

A case of hepatic abscess, penetrating between the skin and the ribs, and opening into the axilla, is related by Portal. (*Anatom Médicale*, t. v, *p.* 304.)

The duration of life after the spontaneous bursting of the abscess into any of the viscera or cavities, is a point of much interest, and one, which it is to be regretted, we have but limited data whereon to base a correct opinion. The following short table sums up all the information which these collected histories afford us on this point.

No. in which the symptoms denoting the bursting of the abscess are noticed.	Cavity or viscus.	Total number of days the patient survived.	Average number of days.
14[a]..........	Lungs	392	28
3[b]..........	Thoracic cavity..	58	19
11[c]..........	Abdominal ,, ..	86	7¾
5[d]..........	Colon	29	6

If this table were allowed to pass without comment, it might lead to a misconception; from the figures as they stand, it would appear that the duration of life, after the abscess has burst into the abdominal cavity, is longer than when it burst into the colon or intestinal canal; this, however, in fact is not the case. A fatal termination, when it bursts into the former site, generally follows in 2, 3 or 4 days, or even in a few hours, as in case 290; but in these histories there are some examples (134, 135,) to show how long life *may* be sustained under this accident—these cases (one of the patients survived 26 days,) are expressly given by Mr. Twining, with this view; in fact, four of these cases (35, 134, 135, 148,) must be regarded as *extraordinary*, and if we omit these four cases, it will be found that the average duration of life after the abscess has burst into the abdominal cavity, is about three days; this termination is not only the most rapidly, but also the most certainly fatal.

The frequency of the co-existence of an ulcerated state of the large intestines and hepatic abscess, has often attracted the attention of pathologists. The subjoined tables will tend to illustrate this point. Omitting from our present consideration the 96 cases in which the condition of the intestines is not mentioned, we have left 204 cases. Of these—

The large intestines were more or less ulcerated in	147	or	72.158	per cent.
,, ,, not ulcerated in	51	or	25.000	,,
,, ,, presented cicatrices of old ulcers in	3	or	1.471	,,
,, ,, ,, abrasions (?) in	3	or	1.471	,,
	204		100.000	

(*a*) Cases 10, 50, 58, 64, 68, 85, 99, 102, 106, 125, 130, 180, 181, 291.
(*b*) Cases 69, 60, 73.
(*c*) Cases 27, 35, 133, 134, 135, 148, 179, 231, 232, 239, 290.
(*d*) Cases 67, 138, 177, 178, 230.

If we further exclude from our calculations the six cases included under the last two headings, we have 198 cases left; and of this number, as we see from the above table, the proportion of an ulcerated to a healthy or un-ulcerated condition of the intestines, is as 74 to 26 per cent.

The locality of these ulcerations, is specified in 170 cases: it was present—

In the colon alone in	...	...	55
In the cæcum alone in	...	...	5
In the cæcum and colon in	...	...	18
{ In the cæcum, colon and rectum	...	...	7
{ Throughout the large intestines	...	...	23
In the colon and rectum in	...	...	8
In the cæcum and rectum in	...	...	1
"In the large intestines," (exact site not given)		...	28
In the lower end of the ilium, the ulceration extending from the large intestines[a]	...	...	13
In the ilium alone[b]	...	...	2
			170

It will be seen from this, that no portion of the large intestines remains specially unaffected by ulceration, when hepatic abscess exists, but I have never met with the record of a case in which the ulceration was confined to the rectum alone, as co-existing with an abscess in the liver.

The ulceration is mentioned as being confined to the ilium alone in two cases, (No. *224*, *249*;) but in both these instances there was other extensive, co-existing disease of the large intestines; in the former, the mucous coat of the colon was prodigiously thickened, smooth and red, resembling muscular tissue throughout; and in the second case, there were a number of small abscesses about the cæcum coli.

Having thus mentioned the fact, that the ilium is in some instances the seat of ulceration in cases of hepatic abscess, we may here briefly state the condition of the other portions of the small intestines under similar circumstances. Ulceration, (excepting in the cæcal extremity of the ilium, and then only when combined with disease of the large intestines,) is very rarely met with in the small intestines, as co-existing with hepatic abscess. I have never met with a single example of this combination.

(*a*) Cases 101, 143, 144, 158, 215, 216, 218, 219, 220, 223, 224, 229.
(*b*) Cases 224, 249.

In 46 cases in which *the state of the small intestines* is mentioned in the preceding cases, they are described as healthy, in 18; more or less congested, or injected, or vascular, in 7; thickened, in 2; inflated, in 1; pale, or pale and flaccid, in 2; of dark bluish colour, in 1; and of an ashy appearance, in 1. The ilium presented patches of engorgement in 2, was thickened and pearly in 1, was softened, pulpy and contracted in 1, and was covered with granular lymph, in 1, in addition to the 15 cases, before mentioned, in which ulceration existed.

The character and extent of the ulceration in the intestines, merit a brief consideration. They are described simply as ulcers, or ulcerations, in 49; gangrenous, sloughing, or sphacelated, in 25; (perforation of the intestines, in 12 of these cases;) extensive, in 20; partial and slight, in 7; in small or large patches, in 5; numerous small ulcers, in 5; superficial, in 3; healthy, healing, cicatrizing ulcers, in 4; ulcers, some of which were either cicatrizing or cicatrized, in 8; round and solitary, in 2; transverse ridges of ulceration, in 2; small follicular, in 2; incipient, in 2; indolent, in 1; small and pale, in 1. The colon was studded with small granular ulcers in 1, and in another (235,) it was covered with small granular points. There were cicatrices of old ulcers in 3, and abrasions of the mucous coat in 3. The colon was in a state of melanosis in one case, (No. 119.)

The extent of the ulceration in the intestines bears very slight, if any, relation to the extent of the suppurative disorganization in the liver; the abscess may be most extensive, whilst the intestinal ulceration is slight; in case 9, there were only a few indolent ulcers in the cæcum, yet the liver had three distinct abscesses, containing four pints of pus, besides several small abscesses in other parts of the liver. Cases 11, 42, 90, 91, &c., may be consulted in support of the same fact. On the other hand, there may be extensive sloughing ulceration of the intestines, and at the same time, the abscess in the liver may be of small dimensions. This is the case in 109, 114, 116, 119, 137, &c.

The Liver. As might naturally be expected, this viscus departs more or less from its normal state in the majority of cases, when abscess is situated in any portion of its substance. Of 132 cases, we find that:—

The liver was enlarged, generally congested and softened in...	113
,, slightly enlarged, or not much above its natural size in	6
,, of its natural, or normal size (61, 75, 76, 127, 171) in	5
,, sound and healthy (167, 237) in	2
,, in a state of cirrhosis (101, 117) in	2
,, in a state of gangrene (5) in	1
,, small and pale, with an irregular surface like citron (224)	1
,, small, light coloured, buff (29) in	1
,, extremely atrophied, being no larger than a hand (286) in	1
	132

The enlargement of the liver, so commonly met with in these cases, is generally associated with a congested and softened condition; to this, however, there are exceptions, as in case 215, when it is reported, "enlarged, dense and fatty," and in cases 219 and 227, when, in addition to the enlargement, the liver was dense, dark, and carneous.

It is rare to meet with abscess associated with a small indurated condition of the liver, and still more rare to find it co-exist with such a degree of atrophy, as is described in case 286, where the liver was as flat throughout as a hand, scarcely exceeding a hand in size.

The weight that the liver attains, when it is the seat of abscess, is often very great; in one case (20) it weighed 8½ lbs.; in another (223) 8 lbs., and in others (41, 58, 59) between 6 and 7 lbs.

The size which it may attain, and the extent of surface it may occupy under these circumstances, is very striking:—thus, in case 12, it occupied both hypochondria, the stomach being altogether concealed and pushed back by the left lobe; in cases 41, 58 and 112, it filled the left hypochondrium; in case 47, it occupied the entire epigastric region, from rib to rib; in case 126, it extended into the left hypochondrium, and downwards below the umbilicus; in cases 139, 144, and 152, it descended into the right iliac region, filling the whole of the epigastric and the right and left hypochondriac regions; and in case 157, it filled the whole epigastrium, completely covering the colon and stomach, so as to prevent any part of them from being seen.

The displacements occasioned by these increased dimensions are often great. In one instance, (No. 8) the left lobe of the liver which was very large, had displaced the stomach, making its long diameter perpendicular instead of transverse, and in another case, it had pushed the colon downwards almost into the hypogastrium.

The liver, when thus enlarged, often encroaches to a very considerable extent, on the thoracic cavity;—thus, in cases 13, 20, 95, the liver was on a level with the 4th rib; in cases 82 and 94, it reached the third rib, and in case 79, it was as high as the 2d rib. Case 41, is peculiarly interesting; the diaphragm was pushed up on a level with the mamma, and through this muscle the abscess had worked its way into the cavity of the pleura, but was prevented discharging its contents into the chest, by a thick deposit of coagulable lymph. It is hardly necessary to remark that such great displacements as these, must give rise to most distressing symptoms.

There is another case, (228,) which tends to show, in a remarkable manner, how such extensive enlargements may render our diagnosis a matter of no small difficulty. The left lobe, in this instance, was the seat of disease; it contained two large abscesses, and from its increased size, it appears to have caused powerful pressure on the abdominal aorta, immediately above the cæliac artery. The prominent symptom was a tumour at the epigastrium, and at this point arterial pulsation was very distinct, although the patient was largely covered with bed clothes; he likewise suffered much from palpitation of the heart. After death, the aorta was found encircled by a broad band of inflammation, (just where the pressure from the enlarged lobe was supposed to have been,) and the surrounding cellular tissue was injected with red gelatinous serum. In case 232 also, the abscess simulated abdominal aneurism.

In conclusion, it may be remarked, that it not unfrequently happens that one portion of the liver may be enlarged, whilst the remaining parts retain their original size;—thus the enlargement appears to have been principally confined to the right lobe in cases 56, 107, 256 and 257, and to the left lobe in cases 2, 10, 50 and 242.

Cicatrices on the surface of the liver are supposed by some to indicate that hepatic abscess had existed at some former period, and that these cicatrices mark the spot through which the contents of the said abscess have escaped. Without denying that after the evacuation of an hepatic abscess, a cicatrix may mark the position of the puncture, (as was observed in case 172,) yet what the real nature of the larger proportion of those appearances termed cicatrices is, appears to be very doubtful. In case 229, thirteen deep sulci were found, on the convex surface, with extensive thickening, and white corrugations resembling scars. Now is it conceivably possible, that thirteen abscesses could have burst into the abdominal cavity, and left nothing to tell of their former existence, but a few scars? Again, in case 230, there was a large "scar" over the gall-bladder, of which the centre formed a deep notch on fissure. Could this have been the remains of an abscess? In case 64, the patient had had an abscess in the liver opened two years previously, yet no cicatrix nor mark of cavity of former abscess could be found;—it should, however, be added, that the liver was in a very softened state, which may account for those appearances, which might have been expected, not being observed. No trace of abscess could be discovered in another case, (255,) although the abscess had been evacuated six months previously.

The real nature of these cicatrices is a matter for future investigation; with our present amount of information, all we can say is, that the existence of a cicatrix, however well marked, cannot be regarded as certain evidence of the existence of hepatic abscess at a previous date. The reader can consult cases 7, 64, 172, 222, 225, 229, 230, 240, 255. It appears to me probable that, in their nature, these so called cicatrices, are allied to the white spots or pearly patches met with on the surface of the heart.

The gall-bladder, although noticed in 46 cases, is only described as healthy or natural in 2; (47, 170;) in all the others, it had departed more or less from its normal state. In one instance, (No. 5,) it was completely disorganized, and removed by gangrene. In 8 cases, it is described as small, contracted, diminished, or flaccid; and in 12, it appears to have been distended or full; in one of these cases, (152,) it had attained the size of the urinary bladder when distended with urine; and in another, (229,) it extended four inches below the inferior border of the liver, and presented a soft elastic tumour, which might easily have been mistaken for an abscess in the liver, pointing externally. It was inflamed in one case, (92,) and covered with a false membrane in two; (129, 137;) and had very thickened walls in two. In one case, (160,) it communicated with the abscess.

With respect to the contents of the gall-bladder, it is almost impossible, in a limited space, to specify the varieties of colour, consistence, &c. The bile is variously described as of an orange colour; pale, straw colour; thick, dark, tar-like; dark, tenacious; a thin fluid; green; green, ropy bile; brownish green; dark, grumous bile; inspissated, &c. &c. The gall-bladder was empty in three cases, (25, 43, 246,) and nearly empty in another, (237.)

A few cases require special notice; thus, in case 47, the gall-bladder contained a large firm coagulum of blood; and in cases 214 and 223, it contained bile and pus. In case 230, there was a large scar, (cicatrix?) over the gall-bladder.

The condition of the mucous coat of the stomach, is mentioned in 38 cases. Of this number, it is reported to have been healthy in 13,(a) and in 4(b) others, it presented some slight changes in colour, but was unchanged in structure. In case 43, the mucous coat was indurated and thickened; in case 44, vascular and softened in parts; in No. 46 and 230, congested; in case 215, dark and corrugated; and in case 218, the stomach was flaccid, with points of ecchymosis. In eight other cases it presented some slight deviations from the normal state. In case 73, it presented some abraded spots, and at other parts it was thickened and mammillated. In only two instances, (No. 75 and 152,) was the mucous coat found inflamed; and in the latter of these cases the abscess was adherent to the walls of this viscus. In cases 1, 80, 152, 220 and 259, the abscess was adherent to the stomach; and in No. 220, it was making its way, by the ulcerative process, through its walls; at this part the mucous coat presented an ulcerated point. In two instances, (241, 243,) the abscess opened into the stomach.

I think that it will fairly admit of a question, whether some of the slighter deviations from the normal state, observable on the mucous surface of the stomach, were not produced by the powerful and irritating drugs, especially mercurials and purgatives, which it was the routine practice to administer with no unsparing hand, whenever hepatic disease was suspected to exist.

The lungs in these cases, present a great variety of conditions; in 36 cases they are reported as healthy or free from disease, in some there were old adhesions, apparently unconnected with the hepatic affection, but these are not to be confounded with others in which some portion of the right lung was adherent to the diaphragm; in these latter cases the adhesions were evidently recent, the result of inflammation set up by the pressure of the liver, and it was by means of these adhesions that the bronchial ramifications communicated with the hepatic abscess. In five cases, (No. 50, 85, 99, 122, 142,) there was a distinct abscess in the lung, communicating with the abscess in the liver, and in another (226), though an abscess existed both in the lung and in the liver, no communication between them appeared to exist. In three cases the lungs contained suppurating tubercles, and in three others they are stated to have been tuberculated. The lungs are reported as collapsed in 10, congested and hepatized in 9, emphysematous in 8, com-

(a) Cases 42, 59, 60, 76, 79, 110, 111, 138, 148, 158, 237, 240, 248.
(b) Cases 78, 92, 94, 97.

pressed in 4, engorged in 6, and atrophied in 3. The degree of atrophy was very notable in three cases; in one, (224), the lung lay flat to the spine, reduced to the volume of a middle sized muscle; in the second, (286), it was no larger than the size of a closed hand, and in the third, (227), it was so small that at first it appeared wanting altogether.

In case 50, the bronchial glands were enlarged, and contained a melanotic deposit, which stained the fingers black.

There was effusion into the thoracic cavity in 19 cases, serous in 4, purulent in 9, sero-purulent in 3, fibrinous in 1, and consisting of serum and lymph in 1. The quantity effused was in some instances very large; in two cases, (86, 227) it amounted to five pints; in one (60) to six pints, and in another (62) to eight pints.

Cases 236 and 288, are examples of the extensive disorganization of the lungs, which is occasionally met in this disease.

Heart. We have notice of this organ in only 26 cases. Of this number, eleven are described as healthy, normal, or not diseased; and in another case (107) the outer surface was more pearly than natural, but was otherwise healthy. The heart was enlarged in 2; somewhat enlarged, with flakes of coagulable lymph on its surface, in 1; pale and flaccid, in 1; flabby, in 1. In one (231), there was hypertrophy of the right ventricle, and in another (157), there was a polypus in the right auricle and ventricle. Pearly opaque patches or "white spots," were noticed on the surface in three cases, (85, 110, 161.) In one instance, the surface of the heart was granular, and of a vermillion colour; and in another, (No. 240,) the substance was generally inflamed and softened, the pericardiac covering thickened by opacities, the encordia of both auricles opaque, and in the right ventricle was an organized coagulum, prolonged into the pulmonary artery. In No. 286, the heart was small and its parietes very thin, and this was associated with extreme atrophy, both of the liver and right lung. In eight cases there was more or less effusion into the pericardium, but this was generally associated with some disease of the heart.

The above data are very limited, but as far as they go, they do not confirm the experience of Dr. Allan Webb, (*Path. Indica, p.* 112,) as to the frequency of the co-existence of endo-carditis and hepatic suppuration.

Kidneys. Of these organs, we have notice in 38 cases; of these, 15 are described as healthy, normal, or free from disease; and 1 was very slightly diseased. They were the seat of yellow degeneration, in 5[(a)]; were enlarged, or enlarged and pale, in 3; small,

---

(a) Cases 77, 78, 88, 93, 110.

and pale, in 2; and congested in 3. In one case, (No. 25,) the right kidney was enlarged and soft, bearing traces of recent inflammation; and in another, (217,) the renal tissue was dark, and engorged. The abscess in the liver more or less communicated with the kidneys in 4 cases;(a) and in one of these, (253,) the right kidney was entirely destroyed.

The three remaining cases require separate notice; in one, (No. 216,) the kidneys had some vascular congestion; and pus was observed issuing from the mammillary processes of the left. In the second case, (No. 218,) pressure of the kidneys showed pus passing from the tubuli uriniferi into the infundibulum, on each side. In the third case, (No. 220,) pressure forced pus from the mammillary processes of the kidneys. It is a little remarkable that these three cases should have fallen under the notice of one practitioner, (Dr. Conwell,) on whose authority they are here given.

The spleen, pancreas, and mesenteric glands, present few pathological appearances worthy of note. Only two cases call for remark in this place, No. 151, in which the pancreas was greatly enlarged and hardened, pressing upon the ductus communis choledicus and other ducts, so as almost to prevent the passage of bile, and No. 237, where the mesenteric glands were much enlarged, one containing in its centre a drachm of pus. In the Appendix is given the numbers of the cases in which these organs are mentioned in the preceding histories.

SYMPTOMS.

The insidious nature of hepatic abscess, and the obscurity which not unfrequently characterises the attendant symptoms, should always be borne in mind by the practitioner; and should be regarded by him as an incentive to unremitting attention, and to the utmost circumspection, when treating cases in which the liver is the seat of disease, and the symptoms, at the same time, are of an anomalous or obscure character.

The amount of constitutional disturbance is so small, in some instances, as hardly to attract the notice of the patient himself; of this we have an example in case 48—this patient, though unwell for some years, was at his duty up to the time of his admission; he had only been in hospital a few hours, when an abscess burst into his lungs; and, when he died ten days subsequently,

(a) Cases 32, 233, 253, 287.

the liver was found converted into four large abscesses, containing in the aggregate, more than three quarts of pus;—one abscess had burst into the lungs, a second into the abdominal cavity, and the remaining two, which pointed externally, were found intact. No. 66, is another case in point: this patient died, after being in hospital only five hours and a half; he was a sepoy, and apparently at his duty till the time of his admission. Dissection showed an immense abscess in the liver, containing above two pints of matter. No. 267, is another case of the same description, the abscess having burst whilst the man was on duty.

A few other examples may be mentioned as illustrative of the obscurity of the symptoms in some of these cases.

In case 5, the symptoms crept on so treacherously, that it was only by watching, cross-questioning, and repeated manual examinations, that the fact of an abscess in the liver was confirmed.

In case 18, the patient *never complained of any pain* in the hepatic region, though "latterly abscess was suspected."

In case 40, the only symptom indicative of hepatic disease was pain in the shoulder; the patient had no pain in the liver, no fulness, no increased heat; he did not wince, in the slightest degree, under pressure over the liver; yet, after death, an abscess was found in that viscus, containing a large quantity of pus.

In case 44, there was, with the exception of cold perspiration and hectic, no evidence of hepatic abscess during life.

In case 215, the patient had a craving appetite, was in excellent spirits, and a short time before death, laughed at the idea of being in danger; after death, his liver was found to contain eighteen abscesses.

As illustrative of the obscurity of the symptoms in this affection, the reader may consult cases 12, 40, 44, 151, 240, 262, 285. When the patient is admitted with dysentery, and hepatic abscess supervenes, the symptoms of the former affection may be so severe, as entirely to mask those of the abscess—this was especially the case in No. 161, 166, 237, &c.

We will now proceed to enumerate the symptoms observed in these cases, and will then add a few observations on some of those which are most prominent or constant.

Table of Symptoms.

No. of cases in which the symptom is noticed.	Symptoms.	The symptom was Present	Absent
173	Pain in the hepatic or epigastric region	153	20
	,, increased by pressure	51	13
	,, increased by full inspiration	23	4
101	Enlargement or fulness of the side, or some evident local sign of hepatic abscess	90	11
84	Vomiting and nausea	74	10
34	Hectic fever	34	..
75	Cold sweats, or profuse or clammy perspirations.	72	3
22	Evening or occasional exacerbations of fever	22	..
74	Prostration, exhaustion, or great debility	74	..
57	Emaciation or loss of flesh	57	..
76	Pain in the right shoulder.	48	24
	,, left shoulder, (No. 1, 241)	2	..
	,, both shoulders, (No. 167, 274)	2	..
63	Cough	59	4
47	Rigors	25	22
41	Thirst, more or less urgent	40	1
41	Appetite, impaired or total loss of	33	8
36	Want of sleep or restlessness	35	1
32	Breathing, difficult and oppressed, (dyspnæa)	32	..
6	,, hurried and frequent	6	..
15	Painful decubitus on the left side	10	5
5	,, ,, on the right side	3	3
3	,, ,, on either side	3	..
2	,, ,, on neither side	2	..
8	Flatulence, flatulent eructations, much flatus.	8	..
11	Œdema, chiefly of the extremities	11	..
9	Much depression of spirits, despondency, &c.	9	..
5	Great languor	5	..
2	Jaundice (No. 198, 220)	2	..
4	Yellow suffusion of the eyes	4	..
3	,, ,, ,, skin	3	..

Symptoms, continued.

No. of cases in which the symptom is noticed.	Symptoms.	The symptom was Present.	The symptom was Absent.
15	Countenance expressive of anxiety, anxious.	15	..
9	" shrunk or collapsed...........	9	..
6	" pale, livid, or parchment-like...	6	..
11	" sallow	11	..
18	Abdomen full, distended, tense.	18	..
5	" tympanitic puffing of.	5	..
3	" flat, inelastic, or very hard........	3	..
1	" supple (118)...................	1	..
3	" general soreness of.............	3	..
4	Abdominal muscles, tenseness of..........	4	..
7	Right rectus muscle, tense................	6	1
1	Swelling of the abdomen after eating (214)..	1	..
4	Burning heat at the epigastrium...........	4	..
1	" " in the palms of the hands (228)	1	..
6	Dysuria or stranguary....................	6	..
2	Retention of urine, or suppression of that secretion........................	2	..
3	Syncope, or a tendency to syncope	3	..
3	Startings in the sleep at night (218, 228, 241)	3	..
1	Cramps in the extremities (No. 227).......	1	..
2	Bitter taste, or clammy state of the mouth..	3	..
1	Clavus hystericus	1	..
2	Pulsating tumour at epigastrium, simulating aneurism (No. 228, 232).............	2	..
7	Headache or vertigo....................	7	..
13	Death was preceded by delirium in........	13	..
6	" " by coma in...........	6	..
1	" " by convulsions in......	1	..

Pain in the shoulder. This symptom has frequently been regarded as diagnostic of the abscess in the liver being situated in the superior part of the right lobe. We shall form a better idea of the correctness of this diagnosis by considering, first the position of the abscess in the 48 cases in which this pain existed in the right shoulder; and then the position of the abscess in those 24 cases, in which it is expressly stated that this symptom was absent.

In the 48 cases, then, in which pain in the right shoulder was present, the abscesses were situated as follows:—

One or more abscesses in the right lobe	12
In the upper and superior portion of the right lobe ...	8
In the upper and outer part of the right lobe	4
In the outer surface of the right lobe	1
In the upper and *posterior* part of the right lobe ...	3
On the concave surface of the right lobe	4
One large abscess on the *concave* surface of the right lobe ...	1
One small abscess on the concave surface of the left lobe (167)	1
One abscess between the right and left lobes	1
Abscesses in both the right and left lobes	1
Abscesses on the concave surface of each lobe	1
On the *posterior* (concave?) surface of the liver	2
One abscess in the centre (deep seated) of the liver ...	1
On the upper and superior portion of the liver	2
Numerous abscesses throughout the liver	1
One abscess on the superior, and two on the inferior surface of the liver	1
Two abscesses in the right lobe, and also a circumscribed abscess between the surface of the liver and the ribs	1
Exact site not mentioned	3
	48

In the 24 cases in which pain in the shoulder was absent, the situation of the abscesses in the liver was as follows:—

Inferior, or lower margin, or border of the right lobe ...	4
One large abscess on the convex surface of the right lobe ...	1
,, ,, ,, upper and posterior part of the right lobe	1
,, ,, ,, ,, outer part of the right lobe...	1
,, ,, in the upper or superior part of the right lobe, only half an inch from the surface	1
One small deep seated abscess in the right lobe ...	1
Abscesses in both the right and left lobes	3
One immense abscess occupying the whole of the left, and part of the right lobes	1
In the upper part of the left lobe	1
Numerous abscesses in the left lobe	1
One large abscess on the posterior surface of the liver ...	1
Numerous abscesses in the liver, particularly in the right lobe	1
Liver studded throughout with small abscesses	3
Abscess deep seated in the liver	2
Site not stated	2
	24

From these statements, we are entitled to draw the following conclusions:—

1. That pain in the shoulder is most frequent when the right lobe is the seat of abscess; but—

2. That abscess may exist in the right lobe without this symptom being present in any degree.

3. That though this symptom is most frequently present when the abscess is situated in the superior or upper portion of the liver, it cannot be regarded as a constant or diagnostic sign.

4. That the pain in the shoulder may be present when the abscess exists on the posterior or concave surface of the liver, or in the left lobe, or when it is deep seated, or when the liver is studded throughout with small abscesses.

5. That the absence of this symptom is no proof that abscess does not exist in the right lobe.

In fine. We are entitled to say that pain in the right shoulder is most frequently present when the abscess exists in the right lobe, especially when it is situated in its upper and superior portion, but its presence no more necessarily implies that the abscess is in this lobe, or in this portion of the lobe, than we are entitled to conclude that this lobe is not the seat of the suppurative process, *because* pain in the shoulder is absent.

Pain in the left shoulder only, is reported as being present in two instances, (No. 1, 241.) In the first case, the abscess was large and solitary, occupying the left lobe of the liver; and in the second case, there were three abscesses, one in the left lobe, and two in the right. These cases are highly interesting.

Pain in both shoulders, was observed in two cases. (No. 167, 274.) In the first of these, dissection showed a small abscess on the concave side of the left lobe; and in the second, the abscess was on the upper and convex surface of the liver, opening into the right lung.

The pain in the shoulder is liable to great variations as to site, intensity, and constancy. With respect to its site, it is described as affecting the top of the shoulder, (10, 64,) the back of the shoulder, (40,) the front, (69,) between the scapulæ, (50,) about the end of the clavicle, (64, 139,) &c. In case 291, the pain extended down the right arm; in case 47, the pain in the shoulder was attended with numbness of the arm and wrist; and in case 69, this numbness was also present, extending to the lower extremity. With respect to intensity, it appears to have been severe, (208,) and stinging, (159,) whilst in others, it only amounted to a feeling of uneasiness. In regard to its constancy, it appears to have been most variable; thus, in some, (141, 196, 211,) it was present only at the outset of the disease, or "at first;" in others, (135, 195, 197,) it was only noticed occasionally; in some, only on coughing, (189,) only on pressure over the liver, (139,) only on inspiring deeply, (64,) &c. These are but specimens of the numerous variations to which this symptom is subject.

Pain in the region of the liver, is the symptom most frequently met with in cases of hepatic abscess;—it is not, however, invariably present, as we see from the above table that 20 cases are mentioned, in which it did not exist. It was increased by pressure in 51 cases, and by a deep inspiration in 23. Other circumstances are mentioned under which the pain in the liver was augmented; as by motion, (16, 213,) by change of position, (141, 230,) by lying on the left side, (36, 79, 85,) by lying on the right side, (56, 91, 139,) by lying on the back, (82, 160,) by coughing, (59,) by the motion of a dooly, (4,) &c. In some cases, the pain was only occasional, there being periods at which the patient was comparatively easy; (14, 54, 163, 197, &c.) in others, it only existed at first, (196, 209, 211, 221, 235,) whilst in another class, (15, 186,) it was most complained of towards the termination of the disease; in the majority of cases, however, pain in the liver formed the most prominent symptom in the early stage of the attack, whilst there was reason to suppose that the inflammatory action existed in the highest degree. When the abscess is fully established, the pain in the liver is not unfrequently modified, or it subsides altogether, (55, 61, 235.) It is extraordinary the size the abscess may attain, without there being any pain in the hepatic region; of this, we have an instance in case 143, where the abscess contained three quarts of pus, and yet there was no pain even on pressure! Cases 125, 142, 151, 215, are other examples illustrating the same fact. The condition of the liver in which pain is most frequently absent, is when that viscus is studded throughout with small abscesses. (Cases 166, 185, 188, 215, 218, &c.) The abscess being situated on the concave surface of the liver, (5,) or deep seated in the parenchyma of the organ, (18,) appears to modify the amount of pain present.

With respect to the character of the pain, it is variously described as severe, (6,) intense, (231,) acute, (90,) lancinating, (16,) dull, (30, 288,) heavy, (148, 213,) dragging, (7,) obtuse, (70,) teasing, (146,) stinging, (159,) steady, &c. In some, the feeling did not amount to actual pain, but was more a sensation of uneasiness or soreness; (219, 228;) in others, it is described as "a stitch," or catching pain in the side; (152;) in others, (13,) as a weight in the hepatic region.

Evident enlargement of the liver, or some other external sign, as indicative of the existence of hepatic abscess, is not present in all cases, although the liver itself may have attained a morbidly enlarged size. From the preceding table of symptoms, it appears that there was evident enlargement of the liver during life in 90 cases, whilst in 11 others, this did not exist. In the majority of cases, the enlargement consisted of fulness, or fulness and hardness, in the hepatic region, (12, 22, 26, &c.,) or of a diffused swelling or tumour at the epigastrium, (31, 100, 105, 291, &c.,) whilst in others, there were some peculiarities well worthy of notice. Thus, in case 11, the right side bulged out, and was conspicuously enlarged, compared with the left side, which appeared quite flat; in case 47, the intercostal spaces were much increased in breath; in No. 74, the right side was elevated, and the nipple was on a lower level than that of the left side; in No. 79, there was bulging of the ribs on the right side, and a want of depression in the intercostal spaces; and in No. 122, there was some fulness, with blue veins meandering over the right hypochondrium.

Increased dulness on percussion affords good evidence of an enlarged state of the liver; this dulness is sometimes very extensive, extending as high as the mamma, the second rib, &c. (See cases 73, 74, 79, 82, 122.)

The signs on auscultation indicating enlargement of the liver, are given in cases 73, 74, 79, 122.

This section would be imperfect without considering briefly a peculiar rhonchial sound, often, if not invariably, attendant upon enlargement of the liver, denominated by Professor Walshe "the hepatic compression rhonchus." It is very frequently found to exist in the hepatic region, in persons having enlarged livers; and though it cannot apparently be regarded as diagnostic of the presence of hepatic abscess, yet it may be of great importance in obscure cases, in determining the existence of enlargement of the viscus. It co-exists with inspiration only; or, indeed, seems to be rather super-added to the sound of inspiration, than to co-exist with it; not commencing until the inspiration-murmur appears almost at an end. It is brought out in a peculiarly slow, drawling, lazy manner, its mode of evolution being in this respect the exact reverse of the crepitant rhonchus of pneumonia. It consists of a variable, but commonly, a great number of excessively fine dry crepiti, rather superficial than deep seated, is rendered audible by forced inspiration only, and may be heard in the front, at the side, and in the back, of the right half of the chest, at or near to, the upper edge of the liver. Its existence is completely independent of any affection of the lung itself, and is never found on the left side, in these cases of liver enlargement. The characters of this rhonchial sound, observes Dr. Walshe, are so peculiar, that a mere tyro in the art of auscultation would be able to distinguish it from all other varieties of rhonchus. Of its mechanism, Dr. Walshe offers the following explanation—the lower portions of the lung pressed on by the enlarged liver, undergo a sort of creasing or condensation, which in ordinary breathing, interferes with their expansion. By forced inspiration, the portion of the lung implicated, will be readily understood to be *uncreased,* and so the series of sounds above described, is produced. This hypothesis is rendered more probable by the fact that it often ceases to be audible for a time, after from one to five or six forced inspirations; the lung seems to require rest and time to be again creased up.

Professor Walshe adds, that he is unable to make any positive assertion, concerning the frequency with which this rhonchus attends on enlargement of the liver; but he affirms that in no single case of notable increase of the bulk of that organ, which has fallen under his observation since he first discovered this rhonchus, has he failed to substantiate its existence. The sound may, it is true, escape detection on one or more occasions, but it is never absent for a series of days. (See *Clinical Lectures, Lancet,* 1849, vol. i, *p.* 525.)

Decubitus. It is very easy to understand that, when an organ, such as the liver, becomes much enlarged, as we have seen the liver does to an enormous size, the pressure exercised by it on the surrounding or contiguous parts, may give rise to more or less pain. From the examination of the above histories, I am inclined to believe that the enlargement of the liver, or of a particular lobe of the liver, has more to do in producing pain when the body is in any particular position, than the mere fact that that viscus contains an abscess, whatever may be its size or position. I have carefully examined the descriptions of the post-mortem appearances, in all the cases in which decubitus in any posture was painful, and also in those which it was free from pain, and I can trace no constant connexion between the symptom and the seat of disease. The adhesions which the liver, when thus enlarged, forms with contiguous viscera, seems to exercise an influence in these cases.

Of 35 cases in which this point is noticed, ten(a) patients could not lie on the left side without an increase of pain, and four others(b) found this the easiest position. Three(c) could not lie on the right side, and three(d) others laid on this side easiest.

(a) 6, 36, 48, 70, 79, 85, 87, 157, 240, 241.
(b) 9, 10, 212, 227.
(c) 56, 91, 139.
(d) 80, 145, 242.

Three[a] could not lie on either side, but were obliged to rest with the head and shoulders much raised; two[b] others, on the contrary, could lie on either side, and one[c] found the back the easiest position. Two[d] could not lie on the back and left side, and another[e] could not lie down at all from a sense of suffocation; in this case, effusion into the pericardium may have given rise to the inability to lie on the back. I cannot otherwise account for the discrepancies here detailed, than by considering them to arise from enlargement of the liver, and the adhesions it had formed to contiguous viscera.

Rigors. These are mentioned as present in 25 cases, and absent in 22. In some cases, (138, &c.) these appear at the outset, and seem to mask the first invasion of hepatic suppuration;—in others, (69, 233,) they are present only towards the end of the disease. In others, (47, 67, 291,) there was only one rigor;—in others, (13, 197,) they appear to have been frequent; in the first of these cases, (13,) they recurred daily at noon. In those cases in which rigors were absent altogether, the proportion of abscesses containing pus or purulent matter, is as large as those whose contents were serous or sero-purulent. From the presence or absence of rigors, we can form no opinion as to the character of the matter, or the extent of the abscess.

Vomiting or nausea, was present in 74 cases, and absent in 10. In five instances, nausea existed without actual emesis; but in others, (55, 105, 90, 141, &c.,) the latter appears to have been a constant or frequent symptom throughout. In some instances, (151, 157,) it was confined to the early stage of the disease; and in others, (114, 119, 140, 162, 231,) it was a prominent symptom in the more advanced stages, and towards death. The matters vomited were of the most various descriptions;—dark, inky fluid; (81;) green matter, like verdigris; (140;) dark, green, bilious matter; (150;) viscid bile, or bilious matter; (162, 166, 231.) In one case, (47) it was a dark fluid, like coffee grounds, which proved to be vitiated blood; and in another, (141,) the vomiting was constant; emesis took place without exertion, and the ingesta were returned nearly unchanged.

Vomiting, in these cases, is undoubtedly a sympathetic affection, and does not arise, as Louis asserts, from inflammation of the mucous coat of the stomach. If the reader refers to a preceding page, where the state of the stomach is considered, it will be seen that in two instances only, inflammation of the mucous membrane is recorded; although, in a few cases, there were some

(a) 132, 137, 159. (b) 81, 151. (c) 141. (d) 13, 127. (e) 142.

deviations from the normal state. When the abscess was adherent to the stomach, as in cases 1, 80, 220, and 234, there was more or less vomiting present.

The position of the abscess in the liver appears to exercise some influence in producing vomiting. This will be seen by the following table:—

	No. of times that the abscess was in each lobe.	No. of times that vomiting was present.	Percentage.
Right lobe	163	37	22.70
Left lobe	16	6	37.50
Right and left lobe	35	11	31.42
Right, left, and middle lobes	1	1	100.00
Left and middle lobes	1	1	100.00
Numerous abscesses throughout the liver	20	6	30.00
Site not stated	50	11	22.00

From this, it appears that a much larger proportionate number suffered from vomiting, when the abscess was situated in the left lobe alone, or in the left lobe and other portions of the liver at the same time. In the ten cases in which vomiting is expressly mentioned as absent, the abscess was, in only one instance, in the left lobe; in seven others, it was in the right lobe, and in the other two, the position is not specified.

Dr. Geddes considers that vomiting is not present when the dysenteric symptoms are urgent, and accompanied by ulceration of the large intestines, excepting in those cases where the bowel complaint occurs along with numerous abscesses in the liver. (See *Clin. Illustrations of the Diseases of India, p.* 354.) This holds good with regard to Dr. Geddes's own cases; (184 to 212;) but from cases furnished by others, no connexion appears to exist between the presence of vomiting as a symptom, and an ulcerated state of the bowels. This may easily be seen by taking the cases of vomiting, as given in the Index, and comparing in each case the condition of the liver and intestines after death.

Cough. That this is a sympathetic affection, and does not arise from bronchitis, (as asserted by Louis,) there can be little doubt, in the majority of cases; but in others, when the liver becomes much enlarged, and, pressing upwards, acts as a mechanical irritant, inflammation of the lining membrane of the bronchi is undoubtedly established in some instances. The cough, which is a sympathetic affection, is a short, hard, dry cough, attended by a tickling sensation in the throat; it is generally worse at nights, and is rarely accompanied by expectoration; or, if so, only by a small quantity of viscid mucus or phlegm.(a) It may continue for weeks or months, with little increase or diminution of the hepatic symptom. (141, 219, 226.)

The Stethoscope will readily enable the practitioner to distinguish between this cough, and that arising from bronchitis.

When the abscess in the liver communicates with the lung or thorax, the cough is generally of a much more severe character, is attended by more or less dyspnæa, and accompanied by a copious expectoration of purulent or muco-purulent matter. The character of the expectoration differs much in individuals; it may be pure pus, or thick white purulent matter; or it may be copious, brick-red, puriform matter; (82, 99, 104;) grey puriform; (96;) purulent matter, mixed with coagula of blood; (48;) viscid, yellow mucus; (73;) purulent matter, tinged or streaked with blood. (60, 142, 212.) In some instances, the expectoration was evidently tinged or mixed with bile, having a yellow bilious colour, and bitter taste. (7, 130, 291.) In all these latter cases, the lower lobe of the lung communicated directly with the abscess in the liver.

The quantity of matter expectorated is sometimes very large; thus, in case 274, the quantity amounted to four pounds in the 24 hours.

Ptyalism or Salivation. Much has been said by various writers on the difficulty of establishing mercurial salivation, when hepatic abscess exists; and a superficial glance at the above cases, might lead the reader to suppose that this difficulty had been overrated. The results of mercury are mentioned in 54 cases; of this number, 18 patients were brought under its influence, or ptyalism was established; 17 had their gums made sore, or ulcerated, but without ptyalism; and in 19, mercury produced no visible effects, except perhaps, increasing the gastric and constitutional irritation. Two circumstances tend to modify these results; first, in those who were salivated, mercury had probably been given early in the disease, whilst inflammation alone existed before the supervention of the suppurative process—and it cannot, consequently, be said correctly, that they had been salivated notwithstanding the existence of hepatic abscess; and secondly, medical men, generally regarding the undoubted fact of salivation under such circumstances as rare, have pointedly mentioned the fact, when it has occurred; whilst another class, entertaining the same opinion,

(a) See cases 13, 41, 43, 72, 73, 79, 98, 100, 141, 145, 219, 226.

have failed to notice the fact of the failure of mercury on the system, as being a circumstance of too common occurrence to merit being specially mentioned.

When abscess has formed in the liver, it is undoubtedly a matter of great difficulty to bring the system under the influence of mercury; of this fact, we shall only mention two illustrative cases, No. 9, in which 210 grains of calomel were given, and No. 20, in which in addition to scruple doses of calomel internally, mercurial frictions were diligently employed, and in both cases, no effect was produced on the sytsem.

In a subsequent part of this paper I shall have to notice the subject of mercury in abscess of the liver, and shall therefore defer any further remarks in this place.

Tension of the right rectus muscle. Much stress was laid by the late Mr. Twining on this symptom; it however appears to be not only not a constant, but not even an ordinary symptom; as far as the above cases are concerned, it is mentioned as being present in five instances, (13, 80, 90, 233, 291,) and absent in one, (64.) It is mentioned in one of these cases, (13,) the right muscle was more tense than the left, "*or rather it became so, on attempting to examine the liver;*" and this I believe to be the true solution of many of those cases, when this symptom has been observed. Dr. E. Impey states, that his experience does not confirm the opinion of Twining on this point. (See *Trans. of the Med. and Phys. Society of Bombay*, vol. vii, *p.* 176.)

Dr. Budd, ("*On Diseases of the Liver,*" *p.* 86,) after remarking that this symptom, when present, is purely sympathetic, observes that it is met with in other diseases besides abscess of the liver; that he met with it in a case of long continued jaundice from closure of the common duct; in a case of cancer of the stomach, when the latter viscus adhered to the liver; and he also quotes a case from Dr. Graves, in which this symptom was noticed when the gall-bladder was inflamed.

Other conditions of the abdomen, are worthy of note. There was fulness and distention of the abdomen in 18, a tympanitic state of, in 5, and general soreness of, in 3. In one case, (214,) there was much swelling of the abdomen only after eating. The abdomen was flat, inelastic, or very hard, in 4; (No. 135, 137, 234, 289;) supple in 1, collapsed and retracted, in 2. In only one case, (291,) is the abdomen described as doughy, and this is a little remarkable, as a peculiar doughy state of the abdomen, is as far as my limited experience goes, a very frequent symptom in these cases. There was general tenseness of the abdominal muscles in four instances, (128, 135, 231, 238.)

The condition of the urine, is mentioned in 45 cases. It was—

High coloured and scanty in	7
,, ,, with thick white deposit in ...	2
High coloured in	4
Scanty in	2
Purulent, containing purulent matter, or a puriform deposit..	6
Red and turbid, (50,) turbid like ale, (230,) turbid without deposit, (242)	3
Copious, and like the decoction of cinchona, (218, 220, 229,)	3
Very dark, (228)	1
Surcharged with bile, (233)	1
Not high coloured (159)	1
Natural, (64, 160, 226,) in 3; free, (71, 225,) in 2 ...	5
Dysuria or stranguary	6
Retention or suppression (25, 134)	2
At first dark, towards death, pale with a thick white deposit (217)	1
At first high coloured and scanty, coagulating slightly when heated, latterly of a deep colour with a white powdery sediment, (291)	1
	45

From this, it appears that there is nothing pathognomonic in the character of the urine, in cases of hepatic abscess. Its most frequent state is high coloured and scanty, or containing a white deposit, commonly considered as purulent or puriform in its nature. It is worthy of remark, that in those cases in which the urine was purulent, (No. 13, 30, 45, 223, 224, 227,) there was no communication between the abscess and the kidneys. In what manner, therefore, was the purulent matter eliminated from the system through the kidneys? During the progress of a case, the urine assumes very different appearances at different times: this is particularly observable in case 227. In case 13, the urine sometimes contained much puriform deposit; but after the abscess had been opened by operation, it became quite clear. This subject is again alluded to, when considering the possibility of an abscess in the liver being cured by the absorption of its contents.

Stools. It is a matter of great difficulty to ascertain, with any degree of correctness, the characters of the stools, in cases of hepatic abscess, in consequence of a practice which prevailed for a long time, (now, less than formerly,) of administering aperients, almost daily, as a sort of regular routine. No one can read through the daily records of one of these cases, such as is given in Annesley, for example, without remarking the extremely different and opposite descriptions of the evacuations, at intervals of a few days. As far as practicable, I have arranged these evacuations in 176 cases, in the following manner:—

Stools, more or less vitiated, deranged, or unhealthy, in ...	46
,, dysenteric	36
Free, regular, natural, feculent	20
Diarrhœa, chiefly colliquative, and towards the close of the case	15
Bowels constipated, requiring purgatives to procure evacuations	6
Stools contained purulent matter	16
,, ,, coagula of blood, or grumous blood ...	15
,, black and watery, resembling coffee grounds ...	6
,, perfectly white, latterly, (case 160)	1
Bowels irregular, sometimes relaxed, at others costive, &c. in	12
,, irritable	3
	176

Great discrepancies are apparent in perusing the preceding collected cases: thus, in some instances, (No. 15, 19,) the bowels were at the outset of the affection, constipated, but subsequently became dysenteric; whilst in others, the stools, which had been dysenteric in the first stage, became much more feculent, and in some quite natural, before the fatal termination. (Cases 11, 157, &c.)

There are two forms of stool, from which an unfavourable diagnosis may be drawn. 1st. Black, watery stools, like coffee grounds, as in cases 47, 162, 213, 215, 218, 230, 237. 2ndly. Stools containing coagula of blood, or grumous blood; these are rarely observed till towards the close of the case; they are recorded in cases 67, 84, 123, 131, 137, 157, 166, 215, 221, 225, &c.

With respect to those cases (a) in which purulent matter was passed in the stools, it was very evident, that in some instances, this depended upon the abscess in the liver opening into some part of the intestinal canal, as in No. 67, 138, 149, 177, 178, &c.; but in others, (17, 30, 32, 41, 58, 84, 89, 148, 271,) no distinct communication was found to exist after death, between the abscess and the intestines, although in some (30, 89,) the abscess was adherent to some portion of the intestinal parietes. In the remaining cases, no apparent communication whatever appears to have existed. The question, how, under these circumstances, purulent matter was passed by stool, remains to be solved by future enquirers.

(a) Cases 17, 30, 32, 41, 45, 58, 67, 89, 138, 148, 149, 177, 178, 230, 271, 291.

The number of stools, in most instances, appear to increase during the night;—this is particularly observable when the hepatic affection is combined with dysentery or diarrhœa.

It is very remarkable, how slightly the fecal evacuations deviate from a normal or healthy state, in some instances, even when the most extensive disorganization has taken place in the liver. Of this we have a striking example in case 79.

The Pulse, in these histories, presents but few points worthy of note. In the early stages of the disease, it has generally been full and soft, accelerated towards night; and in more advanced stages, it becomes irritable, rapid, and contracted. Quickness of the pulse is about one of the most uniform symptoms in cases of hepatic abscess; but, still, exceptions not unfrequently present themselves; as in cases 76, 77, 133, 139, 152, &c. The lowest number of beats in a minute, in any of these cases, is 76; but examples are to be found in which the number was much less; thus, Dr. J. Don, (*Trans. of the Med. and Phys. Society of Bombay*, vol. iii, *p.* 18,) mentions a case in which the pulse was slow and weak, seldom rising above 63, even after unequivocal symptoms of suppuration had taken place; abscess was found after death. Dr. Floyd, (*Ibid*, vol. iv, *p.* 40,) cites another example of fatal hepatic abscess, in which the pulse seldom exceeded 58; these, however, must be regarded as exceptions to a general rule.

The Tongue presents no uniform appearance in this affection; but the description given of it, in by far the larger number of cases, is, furred or loaded at its base or centre, its edges and tip being of a morbidly red or florid hue; it need, however, hardly be observed, that this state of the tongue is not met with uniformly in any series of cases, nor even in a single case throughout its whole course. The smooth shining tongue, regarded by Annesley as indicative of organic disease of the liver, is only mentioned as existing in five cases. A smooth red tongue, "chopped," or fissured with sulci running in all directions, appears to be not uncommon. (152, 167, 217, 222, 224, 291.) One circumstance relating to the tongue should not be passed over in silence; namely, that in some instances, a tongue which had been furred, loaded, and foul at the commencement, and during the early stages of the disease, becomes perfectly clean and natural in the more advanced stages, and shortly before death. This was observed in cases 139, 144, 149, 160, 240, &c.

The Skin presents little worthy of note;—during the early stages, and whilst inflammation ran high, it was generally hot and dry, having in some cases a stinging, (230,) or a harsh and dry (64) feel; whilst in others, (150, 159,) it was greasy and unctuous. On the subsidence of the inflammatory symptoms, the skin appears to become reduced in temperature, and in some instances to be almost natural. As the disease advances, the skin may or may not be above the natural temperature, but it becomes clammy, or covered more or less with cold perspirations, particularly at nights. In 13 instances, it is described as sallow, or very sallow.

SUMMARY

OF

EIGHTY-ONE CASES IN WHICH THE CONTENTS

OF

ABSCESS IN THE LIVER

WERE EVACUATED BY OPERATION.

(The only cases included in this Summary are those occurring in India, and within the present century.)

Case I. *Recovered.*—J. Smith, æt. 36, admitted Jan. 9th, 1839—operated on, Jan. 28th—fluctuation evident—trocar only employed—site, the right side of the lower extremity of the ensiform cartilage—8 oz. of thick, purulent matter drawn off—afforded instantaneous relief—canula left in situ, there being no adhesion between the liver and the abdominal parietes. Discharged April 26th—reported in good health on the 3d of June. *(Dr. E. Mockler, Madras Medical Journal,* vol. i, *p. 336.)*

Case II. *Fatal.*—R. Parke, æt. 34, admitted Feb. 6th, 1839—operated on, Feb. 25th—fluctuation evident—trocar only employed—34 oz. of sanio-purulent matter drawn off—afforded much relief—canula left in situ—discharge ceased on the 28th—trocar re-introduced, March 2d—discharge as on the first occasion—afforded great relief—the discharge having again ceased, the trocar was introduced a third time, on March 7th—about 30 oz. of pus escaped—on the 9th, the discharge being very fetid, a mixture of chloride of soda and water was injected into the sac of the abscess—became much exhausted—died March 14th—17 days after the first operation. Not combined with dysentery.

Autopsy.—Immense abscess in right lobe of the liver—evidently contracted since operation—contained only a few ounces of curdled matter—had been opened at its most dependent and superficial point—it was adherent to the ribs and diaphragm; some bands of effused lymph had formed at the lower portion of the convex surface of the liver. There was no effusion of pus into the peritoneal cavity—traces of former ulceration in large intestines. No. 6 in Fatal Cases. (*Dr. Murray, ibid,* vol. i, *p.* 473.)

Case III. *Fatal.*—Lieut. Bligh, admitted Feb. 6th, 1839—distinct succussion perceptible—operated on, March 8th—trocar only employed—introduced between the 9th and 10th ribs, obliquely, upwards, and inwards—9 pints of thin, flaky, purulent matter drawn off—canula left in situ—afforded much relief—in addition to the purulent matter, air was forced out when the patient coughed—the discharge having ceased, the trocar was reintroduced on the 20th, when a pint of matter was evacuated. On the 21st, the pus was fetid, smelling strongly of sulphuretted hydrogen. Died in a fit of exhaustion, March 22d, 14 days after the first operation. This was a hopeless case, before the operation was performed—all that was contemplated by it was effected—namely, relief of distressing symptoms.

Autopsy.—A large abscess in right lobe of the liver communicated freely with the right lung, which was only prevented from collapsing by extensive adhesions—pleural cavity full of a red serous fluid, of a very fetid odour. The trocar had gone through two folds of peritoneum, and easily reached the abscess, which was distant half an inch from the surface. *Though no adhesions had taken place between the two opposite layers of the serous membrane, not a drop of pus had escaped into the abdominal cavity, nor had any inflammatory effusion ensued at any point.* The abscess was not empty, notwithstanding all the evacuations. The hepatic tissue was livid, and inclined to green. No. 7 in Fatal Cases. (*Dr. McGrigor, ibid,* vol. i, *p.* 476.)

Case IV. *Recovered.*—S. Wilks, æt. 35, admitted March 21st, 1839—operated on March 30th—trocar only employed—gave vent to 1 ounce of very black blood, without any admixture of pus—afforded great relief—trocar introduced a little more anteriorly, gave exit to more black blood, but no pus. On the 5th of April, a long curved trocar, (such as is used for puncturing the bladder, per rectum,) was introduced, and gave vent to 4 ounces of sanio-purulent matter, to the great relief of the patient. The discharge having ceased, the long trocar was again introduced on the 11th, matter became healthy—ceased to flow on the 10th of May. Returned to duty June 7th—was in good health two months after that date. (*Surgeon Wilkins, H. M. 45th Regt., ibid, p.* 479.)

Case V. *Fatal.*—A seaman, æt. 39, no unequivocal evidence of the existence of matter—exploring needle first introduced, at two inches in a right line from the junction of the cartilages of the 7th and 8th ribs—a few drops of purulent matter discharged—external opening then enlarged and trocar introduced—gave exit to 8 ounces of thick healthy pus—afforded much relief, but this was the only benefit—the man died two days after. Not combined with dysentery.

Autopsy.—Liver very large. There were no adhesions anteriorly, except for about a quarter of an inch around the puncture, where there was effused a recent deposit of lymph. The abscess punctured was nearly in the middle of the right lobe; besides this, there were two other abscesses in the right, and one in the left lobe. The sac of the punctured abscess had evidently contracted considerably. No. 12 in Fatal Cases. (*Dr. Mortimer, ibid*, vol. ii, *p.* 225.)

Case VI. *Fatal.*—W. Leg,—dates not given—exploratory needle employed, but without detecting pus—introduced a second time with success—trocar then used, and a large abscess evacuated—he was better for some days, but then became worse, with an increase of hectic symptoms, and he died.

Autopsy.—On dissection, it was found that he had other abscesses. The first puncture had healed, and the second, leading to the cyst of the abscess, had united it to the pleura. "So far as the operation was concerned, it was safe, and unattended with a single untoward consequence." (*Dr. Mouat, ibid*, vol. ii, *p.* 227.)

Case VII. *Recovered.*—J. McEldoon, æt. 38, admitted Nov. 11th, 1839—operated on Nov. 22d—fluctuation evident—*no adhesion between the liver and abdominal parietes*—trocar only used—introduced at epigastrium—2 pounds of brown thin matter escaped—great relief—canula left in situ—for a few days about 2 ounces of greenish bilious matter came away, after which the discharge became gradually healthy—ceased Feb. 19th—embarked for England. He died on the voyage in June, about six months after operation, from another disease. Not combined with dysentery.

Autopsy.—Liver enlarged and dark. *There were no adhesions to any part of the abdominal parietes, except at the point where the puncture had been made; and at this spot, it appeared as if it was attached to the walls of the abdomen, or rather hung from it, by a cord about the size of a small goose quill. On dividing its substance minutely, not the slightest vestige of an abscess could be found, or anything which would indicate such having existed.* Some patches of ulceration and cicatrices in large intestines. No. 255 in Fatal Cases. (*Dr. Everard, ibid*, vol. ii, *p.* 229, and *Dr. Mockler, ibid*, vol. iii, *p.* 392.)

Case VIII. *Fatal.*—J. Gorman, æt. 33, admitted February 8th, 1840—no fluctuation perceptible—operated on March 2d. Dr.

Murray says, "I pushed a trocar into the epigastrium, but only a little blood flowed out; not satisfied with this exploration, I pushed the new exploratory instrument into the liver, behind the middle of the side, between the 8th and 9th ribs, when pus flowed • • • —I then withdrew the explorer, and introduced a large sized flat trocar, by which 8 or 9 ounces of thick, curdy pus were evacuated. When the evacuation was nearly completed, a gurgling of air took place through the canula, apparently from the action of the diaphragm, and a cork was then fitted to the canula, (which was left in situ,) with directions to take it out at mid-day and in the evening, to allow the accumulated matter to escape." On the 5th, the discharge ceased, and Dr. Murray made another exploratory puncture into the liver, but without finding pus. He died on the 13th, 11 days after the first exploration. Not combined with dysentery.

Autopsy.—Recent, but firm adhesions had taken place at the point where the punctures had been made into the epigastrium, and attentive examination could not detect any mark of inflammation in the substance of the gland, around the points punctured—the cicatrization of it was perfect. The liver was much enlarged—the abscess opened on the 2d March, was empty—its inner surface had a dark gangrenous appearance, which extended throughout the course of the wound. Besides this, there were two other large abscesses in the liver, one of which pushed the diaphragm as high as the 4th rib. No. 13 in Fatal Cases. (*Dr. Maclean,* ibid, vol. ii, *p.* 232.)

Cases IX, and X. *Both Fatal.*—Two soldiers in H. M. 55th Regt., died in 1836. "In two cases which terminated fatally in this year, (1836,) the abscess pointed outwardly, and was punctured with a fair prospect of success; but hectic fever and dysenteric purging supervened, and on dissection, other deep seated collections of matter were found on the under surface of the organ, beyond the reach of the knife." (*Dr. A. Shanks' Reports of H. M. 55th Regiment, for* 1836. *Madras Medical Journal,* vol. i, *p.* 243.)

Cases XI, XII, XIII, and XIV. *All Fatal.*—Four soldiers in H. M. 55th Regt., died in 1837. Extract from the Annual Report of 1837. "Four of the abscesses pointed outwardly, and were punctured, but without success—other abscesses having existed in three of them, and the fourth having died from a relapse of dysentery when apparently convalescing." The other three cases appear to have been combined with dysentery, being placed under this heading. (*Dr. A. Shanks, ibid,* vol. i, *p.* 258.)

Case XV. *Fatal.*—J. Randal, æt. 44, admitted April 29th, 1839—operated on May 12th—no mention of fluctuation—flat trocar introduced a little to the right of the ensiform cartilage—19 ounces of pus evacuated—great relief—discharge profuse for some weeks—diarrhœa, and also cough, with muco-purulent expectoration supervened. Died June 21st, 40 days after operation. No. 21 in Fatal Cases.

Autopsy.—The abdominal parietes adhered firmly to the convex surface of the liver at the epigastrium; on separating these adhesions with a knife, the sac of an immense abscess presented itself on the upper surface of both lobes, punctured in the most prominent and superficial part. Besides this, innumerable small abscesses throughout the liver. Some ulceration of the colon. (*Dr. Shanks*, *ibid*, vol. iii, *p*. 33.)

Case XVI. *Fatal.*—J. Varney, æt. 43, admitted May 30th, 1839—operated on July 10th—trocar introduced near the point of the ensiform cartilage—2 ounces of matter evacuated—no relief. Died next day. Combined with dysentery—no mention of fluctuation. No. 19 in Fatal Cases.

Autopsy.—Liver much enlarged, adhering to the diaphragm and ribs—several other abscesses in both lobes, besides the one opened. This last was in the right lobe, and its cavity was found re-filled with coagulated blood and pus. Some lymph had been thrown out at the punctured part, and adhesion of the liver to the side had begun to form. Colon ulcerated. (*Dr. Shanks*, *ibid*, vol. iii, *p*. 32.)

Case XVII. *Fatal.*—H. Woods, æt. 38, admitted Aug. 30th, 1839—operated on Sept. 11th—instrument not specified—gave exit to a few drachms of matter. Died next day. No. 20 in Fatal Cases.

Autopsy.—Liver greatly enlarged—studded throughout with abscesses, from the size of a walnut to that of an orange—the entire substance softened and disorganized—the peritoneal coat covering the convex surface, adhered firmly to the abdominal parietes, and the puncture had been made in the most favourable part, but had perforated only a few of the smaller abscesses. Colon ulcerated. (*Dr. Shanks*, *ibid*, *p*. 32.)

Case XVIII. *Fatal.*—J. Carroll, admitted Sept. 25th, 1839—hepatic abscess apparent—operated on Oct. 20th—trocar used—introduced about an inch below the 10th rib—15 oz. of healthy pus discharged—great relief. Everything went on favourably for five weeks, when the wound assumed a sloughy appearance, with increased and fetid discharge, diarrhœa, &c. Died Dec. 6th, 47 days after the operation. No. 22 in Fatal Cases.

Autopsy.—The surface of the right lobe adhered firmly to the abdominal parietes, diaphragm, and ribs. This lobe was converted into an immense abscess; the whole of its substance quite disorganized, and converted into a mass of thick, sloughy matter, amounting to 8 or 10 ounces. The external opening was surrounded by an elevated sloughy margin, of the circumference of an orange. The abscess also adhered to the colon, which shewed traces of former ulceration throughout. *(Dr. Shanks, ibid, p. 34.)*

Case XIX. *Fatal.*—T. Lancaster, æt. 38, admitted Jan. 8th, 1840—operated on Jan. 26th—instrument not specified—fluctuation not stated. 74 oz. of pus discharged before death, which occurred three days after the operation. Combined with dysentery. No. 23 in Fatal Cases.

Autopsy.—Liver large, adherent to the diaphragm and ribs. The right lobe converted into an immense abscess, which had been punctured at its most prominent part. *No adhesions had taken place at the punctured point. 32 ounces of matter were contained in the abscess, and part of the contents had apparently escaped into the abdominal cavity, causing peritoneal inflammation, and a glueing together of the intestines.* *(Dr. Shanks, ibid, p. 35.)*

Case XX. *Recovered.*—Mrs. Mulligan, æt. 45, admitted April 15th, 1829—operated on May 28th—distinct fluctuation perceptible—an incision 2½ inches long, was made through the integuments and muscles, over the centre of the soft tumour—an abscess was then felt, pointing through the peritoneum, which was laid open with an abscess-lancet to the full extent of the external wound, when upwards of 5 pounds of fetid, greenish, watery fluid, were discharged, mixed with some thick flaky matter—lint was then introduced into the opening, dressing to the wound, and a poultice over the whole—was much relieved. For ten days the discharge continued copious, and then gradually diminished. She improved daily and was discharged well Sept. 22d. Not combined with dysentery. *(Dr. Henderson, ibid, vol. iii, p. 153.)*

Case XXI. *Fatal.*—J. Madill, æt. 37, admitted March 27th, 1840—fluctuation obvious—operated on April 3d. Exploratory needle, and then the trocar employed—two bleeding-cups full of pus discharged—canula left *in situ*, and the abscess continued to discharge for several weeks, in great quantity daily; this having ceased, the trocar was again introduced, and as much pus, drawn off as in the first instance. Died 97 days after the operation. No. 26 in Fatal Cases.

Autopsy.—Liver greatly enlarged, containing numerous large deep-seated abscesses. The trocar had entered one situated at its lowermost edge, which yet contained much sanious pus, and seemed to communicate with the others. Colon ulcerated. (*Dr. Sinclair, Madras Medical Journal*, vol. iii, *p.* 187.)

Case XXII. *Fatal.*—J. Taylor, æt. 32, admitted May 7th, 1840—fluctuation perceptible—operated on June 7th. Exploratory needle, and then trocar, employed—three bleeding-cups full of pus discharged—canula left *in situ*—sudden sinking of the vital powers. Died two days after operation. Not combined with dysentery. No. 27 in Fatal Cases.

Autopsy.—Liver contained numerous large abscesses; one of these, on the convex surface, had been punctured, and entirely emptied of its contents; and another, on the under surface, had burst, and its contents had escaped into the abdominal cavity, causing inflammation, &c. The bursting of this second abscess appears to have caused the sudden sinking. No part of the contents of the abscess which was punctured could possibly have escaped into the abdomen, for the canula remained *in situ* after death, and there were firm adhesions between the liver and the side surrounding the place of puncture. (*Dr. Sinclair, ibid*, vol. iii, *p.* 188.)

Case XXIII. *Recovered.*—J. Crampton, æt. 25, admitted June 10th, 1840—no fluctuation perceptible—operated on June 14th. Exploratory needle introduced its full length into the liver, an incision having been previously made with a lancet—no pus flowed—dossil of lint introduced into the wound, and a poultice applied—no bad symptom followed; on the contrary, the patient seemed to feel better. Seven days after, an elastic tumour presented itself, having the wound in its centre—a trocar was introduced, and six ounces of matter evacuated—canula left in situ—discharge continued up to Aug. 22d—gradually recovered. Seven months after, he was sent to England, convalescent. Not combined with dysentery. He is reported before starting as, "fat, but complaining of lameness and numbness in his right leg." The wound of the trocar was quite healed, but he suffered from uneasiness in his liver. (*Dr. Sinclair, ibid*, vol. iii, *p.* 190.)

Case XXIV. *Recovered.*—W. Squires, æt. 25, admitted April 6th, 1840—no mention of fluctuation—operated on June 1st. Exploratory needle and trocar employed. 10 ounces of healthy matter evacuated—afforded great relief—canula left in situ—discharge continued till July 2d. Not combined with dysentery. Discharged Aug. 21st. Reported in good health in November, but he was subsequently obliged to invalid. (*Dr. Allman, Mad. Med. Journal*, vol. iii, *p.* 192, and vol. v, *p.* 323.)

Case XXV. *Fatal.*—J. Silver, æt. 27, admitted Aug. 1st, 1840—no mention of fluctuation—operated on Aug. 17th. Exploratory needle first used, and then trocar—6 ounces of pus drawn off—great relief—canula left *in situ;* no dysentery. Health remained stationary till Oct. 24th, when the abscess was again punctured, and 2 pounds of pus evacuated at first; and fully 3 pounds more, afterwards. Died of exhaustion, Nov. 4th, 76 days after the first operation, and 10 days after the second. No. 31 in Fatal Cases.

Autopsy.—The right lobe of the liver converted into a mere cyst containing upwards of 7 pints of purulent matter. Strong membranous adhesions had formed, between the convex surface and the abdominal parietes around the sites of the puncture. (*Dr. Allman, ibid*, vol. iii, *pp.* 194, 196.)

Case XXVI. *Fatal.*—F. Henwood, æt. 29; hardness over the right lobe of the liver. Exploratory needle and trocar used. 25 ounces of matter evacuated—great relief—canula left in situ—discharge kept up freely—diarrhœa set in. Died Aug. 6th, 7th day after the operation. No. 32 in Fatal Cases.

Autopsy.—Liver adherent to the diaphragm, and also to the side at the point where the puncture had been made—no matter had escaped into the abdominal cavity. Slight peritonitis in places. The sac of the abscess contained very little matter, and was found adherent to, and communicating with the right kidney. (*Dr. Allman, ibid, p.* 195.)

Cases XXVII, XXVIII, XXIX, XXX, and XXXI. *Fatal.* Case XXXII. *Recovered.*—The particulars of these cases are not given: they all occurred in H. M. 80th Regt., whilst stationed at Quilon, between the years 1813 and 1817, and the simple result, (5 died and 1 recovered,) is stated in a tabular form by Dr. Nicoll, in the *Madras Medical Journal*, vol. iii, *p.* 263.

Case XXXIII. *Fatal.*—S. Smallman, æt. 33, admitted April 18th, 1841—fluctuation not mentioned—operated on May 1st. Exploratory needle and flat trocar used—introduced a little anterior to the angle of the ribs, and below their margins. 2 pounds of pus evacuated—great relief—canula left in situ—accidentally slipt out on May 2d; not replaced. May 15th, the discharge having ceased, the trocar was again introduced, (the integuments previously divided with a lancet,) between the 10th and 11th ribs, at their angles. 8 ounces of pus discharged—again afforded relief—canula left in the wound, but gave great pain—when withdrawn, the portion of it which had been in the abscess was quite black—gradually sunk. Died May 23d, 22 days after the first operation. Not combined with dysentery. No. 41 in Fatal Cases.

Autopsy.—Liver greatly enlarged. The abscess punctured was in the right lobe; it was very large, and lined with false thick membrane. The abscess protruded into the thoracic cavity, but had not burst—the diaphragm was pushed as high as the mamma. *The opening made by the trocar had become converted into a canal formed by effused coagulable lymph.* Other abdominal viscera healthy. (*Dr. W. R. Smyth, ibid,* vol. iii, *p.* 382.)

Case XXXIV. *Fatal.*—J. Lightfoot, æt. 25, admitted April 14th, 1841—fluctuation evident—lancet and flat trocar used. 34 ounces of sanious matter evacuated—immediate relief to the dyspnæa, which was urgent. Died May 11th, 5 days after operation, which was only undertaken as a palliative measure, to relieve pain from impending suffocation, threatened by a suddenly aggravated attack of dyspnæa. No. 42 in Fatal Cases.

Autopsy.—Liver firmly adherent to the diaphragm—the right lobe very large, converted into an enormous abscess—the walls scarcely three lines in thickness, and lined to the extent of two inches with a layer of thick pus, which firmly adhered to it. The opening made by the trocar, communicated freely with this abscess. *At this point an adhesion of a tubular form, connecting the external opening in the integuments with the opening in the liver, was found.* Some pale ulcers in the large intestines. (*Dr. Smyth, ibid,* vol. iii, *p.* 390.)

Case XXXV. *Fatal.*—H. Neale, æt. 22, admitted Jan. 16th, 1842—no fluctuation—operated on Jan. 20th. Exploratory needle used—a small quantity of serous fluid drawn off—afforded relief. Died Jan. 28th, 8 days after the operation. Combined with dysentery. No. 46 in Fatal Cases.

Autopsy.—Liver much enlarged—in the right lobe a large abscess, partially filled with turbid serous fluid—no purulent matter was detected, till the substance of the liver was compressed, when it exuded from the sides of the cavity. Large intestines ulcerated—heart hypertrophied. (*Dr. Mouat, ibid,* vol. iv, *p.* 188.)

Case XXXVI. *Fatal.*—A soldier, in H. M. 54th Regt., admitted June 19th, 1837—fluctuation evident—trocar only used—5 pounds of fetid pus drawn off—great relief—copious discharge daily—hectic progressed. Died quite worn out, 24 days after operation. Not combined with dysentery. No. 49 in Fatal Cases.

Autopsy.—Liver much enlarged, adherent to the diaphragm—right lobe, at the place of puncture, adhering to the parietes of the abdomen. Besides the abscess punctured was another, very large, containing matter of a bright orange colour, as if mixed with bile. (*Dr. Stephenson, ibid, p.* 48.)

Case XXXVII. *Recovered.*—Crampton, H. M. 4th Regt.—admitted Aug. 20th, 1841—fluctuation observed—operated on Sept. 20th—trocar employed—nothing but a little blood escaped, although a probe, more than twice the length of the canula itself, passed down into a cavity—neither was there any pus on the probe when withdrawn. On the 6th day after the puncture, pus appeared; and on gentle pressure being made on either side, pus was freely pumped out. For 10 days, there was a copious discharge—the puncture then gradually narrowed, and healed up shortly after. The man perfectly recovered. Not combined with dysentery. (*Dr. Parry, ibid,* vol. v, *p.* 153.)

Case XXXVIII. *Fatal.*—J. Burton, æt. 34—fluctuation obscure—trocar introduced at the lower margin of the 9th rib—12 ounces of pus drawn off—great relief—died from exhaustion, 8 days after operation. Combined with ague. No dysentery.

Autopsy.—The liver, where the trocar had entered, was not more than ¼ inch thick, and was adhering round the wound to the abdominal parietes, for several inches in all directions, so as effectually to prevent the escape of matter into the abdominal cavity. (*Dr. Dix, ibid,* vol. v, *p.* 212.)

Case XXXIX. *Recovered.*—W. Wynterflood, æt. 24, admitted March 28th, 1842—fluctuation distinct—operated on May 24th. Exploratory needle and trocar employed—matter forcibly ejected—3 pints evacuated—canula left *in sitû*—immediate relief—discharge ceased Sept. 7th—left hospital Oct. 11th. Perfect recovery. (*Dr. Anderson, ibid,* vol. vi, *p.* 85.)

* Case XL. *Fatal.*—J. Baker, æt. 37, admitted March 17th, 1840—operated on April 5th,—trocar only employed—6 ounces discharged on operation, and from 2 to 4 ounces daily, to the

---

* Note.—This and the following seventeen cases, are taken, slightly abridged, from "A Return shewing the Results of the Operation for Puncturing Hepatic Abscesses," in the 6th vol. of the *Madras Quarterly Medical Journal.* It is a very important document; but its value is much invalidated by the fact, that the same case has, in several instances, been repeated; this has been overlooked by the Editors. As the Return at present stands, it is calculated to mislead a casual or superficial enquirer.

period of his death. Combined with dysentery. Died June 17th, 73 days after the operation. No. 8 in Fatal Cases.

Autopsy.—Abscess occupied the whole of the left lobe of the liver, protruding into the thorax—only prevented discharging its contents by a thin barrier formed by the diaphragm. Colon ulcerated. *(H. M. 94th Regt.)*

Case XLI. *Fatal.*—J. Lewsey, æt. 22, admitted May 30th, 1840—operated on Sept. 13th. Exploring needle introduced twice—small incision then made with the knife through the skin, then punctured with a trocar—16 ounces of matter discharged. Combined with dysentery. Died Sept. 23d, 10 days after the operation. No. 28 in Fatal Cases.

Autopsy.—One large abscess in right lobe of the liver, that punctured, contained only a little pus. The first puncture with the needle had not been deep enough to reach it. There were slight adhesions around the puncture where the trocar had been introduced. Some cicatrices of ulcers in large intestines. *(H. M. 94th Regt.)*

Case XLII. *Fatal.*—W. Condy, æt. 19, admitted Dec. 27th, 1840—operated on Jan. 29th, 1841—external tumour on the right side opened with a lancet—about 8 ounces discharged every 24 hours. Combined with dysentery. Died 26th April, 88 days after the operation. No. 29 in Fatal Cases.

Autopsy.—Liver small, adherent strongly to the ribs, to the extent of several inches round the wound; under this was a large cavity containing pus, the fistulous opening of the wound communicating freely with it. There were other abscesses in the right lobe. *(H. M. 94th Regt.)*

Case XLIII. *Fatal.*—D. Jobson, æt. 21, admitted Oct. 25th, 1841—operated on Nov. 26th—trocar only employed—6 ounces drawn off. Not combined with dysentery. Died the day after the operation. No. 34 in Fatal Cases.

Autopsy.—Liver very large, studded throughout, and on both surfaces, with numerous abscesses. *(H. M. 94th Regt.)*

Case XLIV. *Fatal.*—J. McGill, æt. 25, admitted Dec. 29th, 1841—operated on March 24th, 1842—small incision made through the skin, under the cartilaginous extremities of the 8th and 9th ribs, and a small trocar introduced—30 ounces of matter drawn off. Not combined with dysentery. Died April 2d, 10 days after the operation. No. 250 in Fatal Cases.

Autopsy.—A superficial abscess in right lobe, had been punctured; it was adherent to the abdominal parietes, and also to the colon; it contained 12 ounces of pus. There was another abscess in the left lobe. *(H. M. 94th Regt.)*

Case XLV. *Fatal.*—J. Blincoe, æt. 30, admitted Oct. 19th, 1842—operated on Nov. 3d—trocar only employed—19 ounces evacuated; free discharge daily till death. Not combined with dysentery. Died 18th Nov., 16 days after the operation. No. 259 in Fatal Cases.

Autopsy.—Liver much enlarged, adherent firmly to the diaphragm, and also to the stomach. The abscess punctured was in the left lobe, and was making its way by ulcerative absorption through the coats of the stomach. The right lobe studded with yellow patches. *(H. M. 94th Regt.)*

Case XLVI. *Fatal.*—J. Wake, æt. 26, admitted May 5th, 1842—operated on May 31st—trocar only employed—4 ounces evacuated; discharge continued June 16th; left hospital under observation Aug. 22d; re-admitted Nov. 6th, with diarrhœa. Died Nov. 12th, 164 days after the operation. Combined with dysentery. No. 249 in Fatal Cases.

Autopsy.—Several abscesses in the right lobe, and one in the left, containing flaky, pale yellow pus. The liver was much enveloped in adhesions, in which the colon, stomach, and spleen were included. There was also a collection of matter between the left lobe and the stomach. *(Dr. Thompson, H. M. 94th Regiment.)*

Case XLVII. *Recovered.*—Mrs. J——, European, private patient, æt. 40, admitted March 3d, 1840—two operations were performed on the 3d and 13th of April. Exploratory needle used in the first operation—no pus flowed; second operation trocar employed—10 ounces of pus discharged. Combined with diarrhœa. Recovered in June, 1840—returned to her usual avocations. *(J. Shaw, Esq., Madras Medical Establishment.)*

Case XLVIII. *Fatal.*—Andiappen, æt. 37, admitted April 27th, 1843—operated on April 30th. Exploratory needle first employed, then the trocar—8 ounces of pus discharged. Died May 28th, 30 days after the operation. No. 256 in Fatal Cases.

Autopsy.—Right lobe of the liver very large, containing at its anterior border the abscess which had been punctured; it was nearly empty, but the sac itself was black and sloughy, and communicated with a larger sac which was filled with curdy matter, but not in a sufficiently fluid state to pass into the punctured sac. The walls of this abscess were also dark and sloughy. *(J. Shaw, Esq.)*

Case XLIX. *Fatal.*—Jackson, æt. 34, admitted March 19th, 1844—operated on April 19th—trocar employed—32 ounces of matter evacuated. *When the plug was withdrawn from the wound, for the purpose of emptying the sac, on the evening of the 20th, (35 hours after the operation,) about 12 ounces of dark coloured pus were evacuated, and there followed about 4 ounces of arterial blood mixed with pus.* The patient became very low, and died two hours after, (37 hours after the operation.) On no other occasion when the sac was emptied did blood accompany the contents of the abscess. No. 258 in Fatal Cases.

Autopsy.—Liver much enlarged, pushing the lung as high as the 4th rib. The greater portion of the right lobe consisted of a sac, the walls of which were formed principally by the peritoneal covering. Notwithstanding the large quantity of fluid evacuated three hours before death, the sac contained much purulent matter, with several large coagula; the hæmorrhage had been from a small vessel, at the floor of the abscess near the transverse fissure. There were some old ulcers in the cæcum. (*J. Shaw, Esq.*)

Case L. *Fatal.*—G. E., æt. 24, admitted Dec. 2d, 1843—operated on Dec. 19th. Exploratory needle first used, then the trocar—8 ounces of pus discharged. Died on the following day, Dec. 20th. No. 257 in Fatal Cases.

Autopsy.—Right lobe of the liver much enlarged, containing a large abscess; (the one punctured;) it was filled with thin pus, and was adherent for some extent to the abdominal parietes. (*J. Shaw, Esq.*)

Case LI. *Fatal.*—D. Parrott, æt. 39, admitted July 9th—operated on 23d. Exploratory needle first used—trocar employed—quantity evacuated not stated. Combined with dysentery. Died July 24th, the day after operation.

Autopsy, not allowed by friends. (*Ibid.*)

Case LII. *Fatal.*—T. Darknell, æt. 28, admitted Sept. 15th, 1843—operated on Oct. 21st. Exploratory needle used—trocar employed—9 pints drawn off. Not combined with dysentery. Died, from exhaustion produced by the excessive discharge, 5th Nov., 15 days after the operation. The canula which was left in the wound, was quite black when withdrawn from the abscess. No. 248 in Fatal Cases.

Autopsy.—Liver large, studded with small abscesses; in the right lobe, one large abscess containing 3 pints of sero-purulent matter. The liver adhered to the abdominal parietes at the point where the puncture had been made. No matter escaped into the abdominal cavity. (*Surgeon J. P. Grant.*)

Case LIII. *Fatal.*—C. Hopkins, æt. 22, admitted 12th Nov., 1841—operated on Dec. 10th—knife and trocar employed; 16 ounces drawn off. Combined with dysentery. Died Dec. 15th, 5 days after the operation. No. 247 in Fatal Cases.

Autopsy.—A large abscess in the right lobe; sac partially emptied of its contents. Colon ulcerated. (*Dr. Dempster, H. M. 21st Regt.*)

Case LIV. *Fatal.*—Capt. H., admitted Dec. 3d, 1840—operated on Jan. 1st. Exploratory needle used—abscess-lancet employed—2 pints drawn off. Not combined with dysentery. Died 6th Jan., 5 days after the operation. No. 260 in Fatal Cases.

Autopsy.—Besides the abscess opened, there were four other large abscesses in the liver. (*Dr. J. Anderson, Mad. Med. Estab.*)

Case LV. *Fatal.*—J. McDonald, æt. 25, admitted May 2d, 1841—operated on July 25th. Exploratory needle and trocar employed—24 ounces evacuated. Combined with dysentery. Died July 29th, 4 days after the operation. No. 248 in Fatal Cases.

Autopsy.—Liver adherent to the side, and also to the colon. The abscess had been punctured about its middle; and from the extensive adhesions around the puncture, no effusion into the peritoneum could possibly have occurred. The abscess had no distinct capsule—contained some dark, yellow, offensive matter—had evidently contracted since it was punctured. Colon ulcerated. (*Dr. J. Anderson.*)

Case LVI. *Fatal.*—W. Quinlow, æt. 27, admitted April 21st, operated on June 20th. Lancet used—no pus. Exploratory needle and lancet used July 28th—16 ounces evacuated. Died Aug. 8th, 11 days after the operation. No. 249 in Fatal Cases.

Autopsy.—The punctured wound was adherent by its edges to the surface of the liver; the abscess opened was between the right and left lobes, and its walls were composed of dense parenchymatous tissue; the right lobe thickly studded with abscesses. The ilium ulcerated, and abscesses about the cæcum coli. (*Ibid.*)

Case LVII. *Fatal.*—S. Shaw, æt. 24, admitted May 29th—had copious muco-purulent expectoration—knife used—operated on Oct. 21st—2 pounds, 6 ounces of pus evacuated—copious discharge daily, sometimes mixed with bile. Died 2d Nov., 12 days after the operation. No. 246 in Fatal Cases.

Autopsy.—Liver adherent to diaphragm and side. In the right lobe were two abscesses; the cyst of the punctured one had evidently much shrunk, and could not contain half the quantity of pus first withdrawn from it; a quantity of pure looking bile occupied one side of it; the gall-bladder empty—it had been punctured in its very centre. The sac was moderately thick, and adhered firmly all around the puncture. Some old ulcerations in the colon.

Case LVIII. *Fatal.*—J. Wells, æt. 26, admitted 18th July, 1844—operated on Aug. 1st—trocar employed—2 ounces of pus drawn off; diarrhœa. Died the day following the operation.

Autopsy.—Liver very large—right lobe formed the cyst of a large abscess, containing 3 pints of very thick pus; the abscess communicated with the right lung. Peritoneum adherent around the puncture. No. 261 in Fatal Cases. (*Mad. Med. Journ.*, vol. vi.)

Case LIX. *Fatal.*—An European, æt. 21, admitted Sept. 14th—operated on Sept. 20th—fluctuation evident—lancet employed—some pus drawn off—quantity not stated—afforded no relief. Died Sept. 22d, two days after the operation. Not combined with dysentery. No. 67 in Fatal Cases.

Autopsy.—Liver much enlarged. The left lobe was one large abscess, from which an opening had taken place into the colon, (this apparently occurred before the abscess had been punctured,) the liver was adherent to that viscus. (*Trans. of the Med. and Phys. Society of Calcutta*, vol. v, *p.* 426.)

Case LX. *Fatal.*—G. Lee, æt. 27, simply stated. "Abscess opened, and matter discharged"—hectic progressed—convulsions preceded death in Nov. 1830, having been in hospital 88 days. Not combined with dysentery. No. 201 in Fatal Cases.

Autopsy.—Abscess solitary in the outer part of the right lobe, penetrating between the ribs to the skin. Intestines healthy. (*Dr. Geddes, ibid*, vol. vi, *p.* 342, and in *Clin. Illustrations of the Diseases of India*, *p.* 317.)

Case LXI. *Recovered.*—Capt. N., dates not given—fluctuation evident—incision $2\frac{1}{2}$ inches long over the tumour, carried down to peritoneum—abscess-lancet used—a quart of flaky matter, and some clots of blood evacuated—wound filled with lint—bandages and compress used—discharge continued free and copious; took a sea voyage; returned in perfect health. Not combined with dysentery. (*Mr. Annesley, Diseases of India*, vol. i, *p.* 656.)

Case LXII. *Recovered.*—An European woman, æt. 25, admitted Aug. 19th, 1819—fluctuation evident—incision over the tumour down to the peritoneum—abscess-lancet employed—6 pounds of green watery fluid, with thick, flaky, ropy matter discharged—cavity filled with lint—covered with a poultice—afforded much relief—discharge continued for 16 days; well six weeks after; left Madras 8 months after in good health. (*Annesley, ibid,* vol. i, *p.* 568.)

Case LXIII. *Fatal, but with temporary benefit.*—Capt. E., admitted March 13th, 1823, expectorating pus and mucus—obscure fluctuation—incision 3 inches long between the 10th and 11th ribs—scalpel used—16 ounces of curdled pus evacuated—much relief—wound filled with lint—matter continued to flow—went on board ship 9 days after operation, in order to avoid the hot season; had a relapse. Died—date unknown. Not combined with dysentery. No autopsy given. (*Annesley, ibid,* vol. i, *p.* 659.)

Case LXIV. *Fatal.*—Lieut. S., admitted Aug., 1820—fluctuation evident, operated on Sept. 13th—instrument used not stated—1 pound of thick white pus discharged—dyspnæa relieved at once; felt easier. Died 5 or 6 hours after the operation. Not combined with dysentery. No. 159 in Fatal Cases.

Autopsy.—Five large abscesses in right lobe of the liver—the one which was opened was separated from another of equal size only by a small membranous septum. The left lobe and other viscera healthy. (*Annesley, ibid,* vol. i, *p.* 664.)

Case LXV. *Fatal.*—J. Gambell, æt. 23, admitted July 1st, 1820—operated on July 22d—incision 2 inches long over the tumour—abscess-lancet used—2½ pounds of matter came out with much force—matter at first green, watery, with flakes of pus—afterwards healthy pus, streaked with blood, and intermixed with a quantity of green bile—greenish copious discharge continued—he became delirious, and died on the 27th, 5 days after the operation. Not combined with dysentery. No. 160 in Fatal Cases.

Autopsy.—A large abscess occupied the whole of the left, and part of the right lobe—it communicated with the gall-bladder. The ducts were impervious, being involved in the adhesive inflammation of the parts forming the walls of the abscess; and the bile was therefore either retained in the abscess, or discharged by the wounds. The other viscera healthy. (*Annesley,* vol. i, *p.* 665.)

Cases LXVI, and LXVII. *Both fatal.*—The particulars of these cases are not given. Mr. Twining, on whose authority they are inserted, simply stating, that since the first edition of his work on the Diseases of Bengal, he has twice opened abscesses of the liver, but in each the result was unsuccessful. (*Twining, "Diseases of Bengal,"* vol. i, *p.* 302, *2d Edition.*)

Case LXVIII. *Recovered.*—Particulars not given. Mr. Twining mentions the case, and merely says that the opening, by incision, (lancet?) was near the epigastrium. The patient lived many years after, and died of some disease unconnected with liver affection.

Autopsy.—Adhesions were found on the convex surface of the liver anteriorly, and an extensive, thick, fibrous structure, occupying a space at that part of about three inches in extent, and nearly half an inch thick. The liver was rather small, of a livid or rather brownish colour, mottled internally. (*Twining, ibid, p.* 302.)

Case LXIX. *Fatal.*—Particulars not given—result only stated. The patient was a Trooper in the Bombay Horse Artillery, and died in 1839. (*Trans. of Med. and Phys. Society of Bombay,* vol. iv, *p.* 57.)

Case LXX. *Fatal.*—W. Harris, æt. 23, admitted Oct. 10th, 1841—fluctuation felt—operated on Dec. 15th—instrument not specified—brick-red, puriform discharge, and air passed from the wound. Died Feb. 1st 1842, 42 days after the operation. Not combined with dysentery. No. 99 in Fatal Cases.

Autopsy.—The opening between the 7th and 8th ribs gangrenous. The integument, and intercostal muscles in a state of sphacelus-caries of the 7th rib. The abscess communicated with a small abscess in the right lung. There were old adhesions of the surface of the liver. (*Dr. Morehead, ibid,* vol. vii, *p.* 47.)

Case LXXI. *Recovered.*—J. Lewis, æt. 26, admitted May 13th, 1847—distinct fluctuation—small incision made May 22d—profuse discharge of pus—immediate relief—all bad symptoms disappeared—discharge very copious till July, when it finally ceased Aug. 9th—left hospital well. He was in excellent health five years after. (*M. Stovell, Esq., ibid,* vol. i, N. S. 1851-52, *p.* 162.)

Case LXXII. *Fatal.*—J. Blundell, æt. 25, admitted Dec. 10th, 1848—distinct fluctuation—opened by a small incision Jan. 10th—much pus evacuated—very copious discharge continued—gradually sunk. Died Feb. 21st, 41 days after the operation. No. 172 in Fatal Cases.

Autopsy.—Liver large. The cavity of the abscess nearly filled up, and the incision which had been made into it had united, and was marked by a cicatrix at the anterior surface of the right lobe of the liver. Colon sphacelated. (*M. Stovell, Esq., ibid, p.* 163.)

Case LXXIII. *Fatal.*—Maria Duart, æt. 27, several times in hospital—re-admitted June 6th, 1848—tumour in the right dorsal region, over the angles of the 7th and 8th ribs; opened; (date or instrument used not mentioned.) There was considerable discharge of pus traceable to abscess in the liver—discharge copious—gradually sunk. Died Aug. 1st. No post-mortem. No. 173 in Fatal Cases. (*M. Stovell, Esq., ibid, p.* 164.)

Case LXXIV. *Fatal.*—G. Davis, æt. 26, admitted Nov. 18th, 1849—fluctuation evident—operated on Dec. 1st—instrument used not stated—22 oz. of pus streaked with blood evacuated—temporary improvement—the discharge became copious—exhaustion extreme. Died Dec. 14th, 13 days after the operation. No. 174 in Fatal Cases.

Autopsy.—Liver greatly enlarged. The abscess occupied the whole of the right lobe; and still contained a large quantity of pus. The other abdominal, and the thoracic viscera normal. (*M. Stovell, Esq., ibid, p.* 164.)

Case LXXV. *Fatal.*—T. Hewett, æt. 37, admitted Dec. 19th, 1850—fluctuation distinct—opened by lancet, Dec. 24th—several ounces of pus evacuated—much relief for a day or two—gradually sunk. Died Jan. 3d, 10 days after the operation. No. 175 in Fatal Cases.

Autopsy.—Liver enlarged—in the right lobe a large abscess containing little pus, and communicating with the incision which hade been made—adhesive inflammation had taken place between the surface of the liver and the abdominal parietes, at the spot which had been opened; thus none of the contents of the abscess had escaped into the peritoneal sac. Small patches of ulceration in colon. (*M. Stovell, Esq., ibid, p.* 165.)

Case LXXVI. *Fatal.*—J. Carroll, æt. 20, admitted July 22d, 1851—fluctuation evident—opened by incision (lancet) Sept. 3d; a large quantity of pus evacuated; did not improve—hectic sweats—exhaustion. Died Sept. 27th, 24 days after the operation. No. 176 in Fatal Cases.

Autopsy.—Adhesion had taken place between the hepatic and parietal surfaces—an abscess in the right lobe containing 8 oz. of yellow pus—the abscess walls uneven, rough, and indurated. Colon ulcerated throughout. (*M. Stovell, Esq., ibid, p.* 166.)

Case LXXVII. *Recovered.*—J. W., æt. 21, admitted April 29th, 1851—fluctuation evident—operated on June 28th—trocar employed—10 ounces of pus evacuated—canula not left in the wound, but a strip of lint introduced with the end hanging out; discharge continued free till Aug. 5th. Left hospital Oct. 1st; returned to his duty. (*Dr. F. S. Arnott, Bombay Establ., Trans. of the Med. and Phys. Society of Bombay*, No. 1, N. S., *p.* 52.)

Case LXXVIII. *Fatal.*— ——, admitted Dec. 31st, 1831—diffused pulsating tumour at epigastrium—opened by small incision Jan. 24th—4½ ounces of fluid of a brick-dust colour, with flakes of pus, evacuated. "Membranes protruded, which were correctly supposed to be the peritoneal coat" (?) great debility came on. Died Feb. 2d, 8 days after the operation. No. 228 in Fatal Cases.

Autopsy.—A slough some inches in diameter encircled the wound, sloughed membranes protruded though the centre—communicated with a superficial abscess in the right lobe, which opened by a fistulous opening into a deep seated abscess. *Some portion of the pus, &c., had escaped into the abdominal cavity;* the remaining portions were retained by adhesions. The wording of the description is very obscure. (*Dr. Conwell, " On the Liver," p.* 521.)

Case LXXIX. *Fatal.*—C. Harrington, æt. 33, admitted Oct. 8th—fluctuation distinct—operated on Oct. 28th—incision, an inch long, over the tumour—trocar used—17 ounces of healthy pus withdrawn—immediate relief—canula left in situ, secured by bandages, straps, &c.—discharge, which had a yellow bilious hue, continued—became very weak. Died Oct. 30th, 2 days after the operation. Not combined with dysentery. No. 241 in Fatal Cases.

Autopsy.—Firm adhesions between the liver and the abdominal parietes—the abscess opened was as large as a man's fist, and perfectly empty. There were also two other abscesses; one of which had burst into the duodenum, and the other into the stomach. (*Dr. J. Jackson, in Webb's Pathologia Indica, p.* 290.)

Case LXXX. *Fatal.*—History given as follows:—In this case there was an abscess in the epigastrium of small size, which on being opened, gave exit to 40 ounces of matter; a catheter was introduced to ascertain its extent, &c., when it was found that *the abscess communicated with the cavity of the pericardium,* and that the pulsation of the heart pushed the instrument aside. Post-mortem examination shewed that there was an abscess in the liver of small size, which communicated with the pericardium, and this had formed an external tumour at the epigastrium. About a pint of matter in the left pleura. (*G. C. Rankin, Esq., in Webb's Path. Indica, p.* 231.)

Case LXXXI. *Fatal.*—J. Russel, æt. 24, admitted Dec. 9th, 1843—seton inserted, and an incision made down to the peritoneum, Dec. 26th—trocar introduced Jan. 3d—indistinct fluctuation—44 ounces of thick purulent matter withdrawn—copious discharge, averaging 8 ounces daily—latterly ill-conditioned, fetid, serous—he became delirious, and died Jan. 11th, 8 days after the operation. No. 242 in Fatal Cases.

Autopsy.—Liver enlarged—the aperture made by the trocar led to an immense abscess, that occupied nearly the whole of the left side of the liver; it contained a large quantity of matter, mixed up with sloughy shreds—the substance around it was soft, and gave way to slight pressure. Rather less than $\frac{1}{4}$ of an inch had been penetrated by the trocar in opening the abscess—several small abscesses in the right lobe. The other abdominal, and the thoracic viscera healthy. *(Dr. F. Anderson, in Webb's Pathologia Indica, p.* 120.)

REMARKS ON THE PRECEDING OPERATIONS.

The proportion of Recoveries and Deaths, in these 81 cases, in which the contents of the abscess were evacuated by operation, is as follows:—

Recoveries	15[a]	or	18.519	per cent.
Deaths	66	or	81.481	per cent.
	81		100.000	

This proportion of recoveries, small as it is, I fear, is overrated, as it is a practice with some medical men, to give prominence to successful cases, and to bury in oblivion those which prove unsuccessful. It is a practice alike unphilosophical and culpable—but easily comprehensible—no one likes to be the herald of his own failures.

Duration of Life after the Operation, in 47 instances:—

Died the same day	1
,, the following day	7
,, from the 2d to the 5th day ...	10
,, ,, 6th ,, 10th day ...	9
,, ,, 11th ,, 15th day ...	6
,, ,, 16th ,, 20th day ...	2
,, ,, 21st ,, 30th day ...	4
,, ,, 31st ,, 40th day ...	1
,, ,, 41st ,, 50th day ...	3
,, ,, 51st day and upwards..	4
	47

The total number of days of life after operation in these 47 cases, is 842; giving an average of about 18 days to each case.

(a) *Recoveries.* Cases i, iv, vii, xx, xxiii, xxiv, xxxii, xxxvii, xxxix, xlvii, lxi, lxii, lxviii, lxxi, lxxvii.

The circumstances which appear to have induced or hastened a fatal termination, may be ranged as follows:—

The presence of other abscesses in liver besides the one opened	19
A combination with dysentery	17
Gangrenous or sloughing condition of the abscess walls(a) &c.	4
Abscess communicating with the lung, (iii, lviii) ...	2
,, ,, with the colon, (lix)	1
,, ,, with the pericardium, (lxxx) ...	1
Two other abscesses opening spontaneously, (lxxix) ...	1
Another abscess bursting into the abdominal cavity subsequent to the operation, (xxii)	1
Impervious state of the hepatic ducts, delirium, (lxv) ...	1
Escape of matter through the puncture into the abdominal cavity, causing excessive inflammation, (xix, lxxviii) ...	2
Abscess making its way by ulcerative absorption through the coats of the stomach, (xlv)	1
Hæmorrhage into the sac of the abscess, (xlix)	1
	51

Death was preceded by great exhaustion, in	6
,, ,, hectic fever, cold sweats, &c. in ...	5
,, ,, diarrhœa, (colliquative) in ...	4
,, ,, delirium, in	2
,, ,, convulsions, in	1
The patients gradually sank, or the symptoms progressed unchecked, in	6

In none of the fifteen cases of recovery does the hepatic affection appear to have been combined with dysentery; in some, this is distinctly stated; in others, it is an inference drawn from the history of the case, the bowels being reported as regular, torpid, and the stools feculent, &c.

The instrument employed, is specified in 58 instances. It should be observed before proceeding further, that when in the history of a case, it is stated that the abscess was "opened by incision," or words to that effect, it has been assumed that the instrument employed was a lancet, or scalpel, or some *cutting* instrument, in contradistinction to the trocar, &c. Thus we find that the trocar only, was used in 23 cases; the exploratory needle first, and subsequently the trocar in 19, and the lancet or scalpel in 16 cases. The following short table shows the ratio of mortality with reference to the instrument employed.

(a) viii, xviii, xlviii, lxx.

Instrument.	No. of Cases.	Deaths.	Recoveries.	Per centage of Deaths to Cases.	Proportion per cent of Recoveries to Deaths.
Trocar only.	23	18	5	78.260	27.777
Exploratory needle first, and subsequently the Trocar ..	19	15	4	78.942	26.666
Lancet, or "by incision"	16	11	5	68.750	45.454

From this, it appears that the proportion in every point of view, is in favour of the lancet, as an evacuating instrument in these cases; but the data here given are on too limited a scale to admit of its being assumed, as an established fact, that the lancet is either the best or the most successfully employed instrument for opening hepatic abscesses. I believe that such an opinion is not in accordance with the experience and observation of most Indian practitioners; but the figures, as given above, are entitled to consideration, and they should teach us, at least, not to *condemn* the use of the lancet in cases of this kind.

The proportion of cases of hepatic abscess which hold out a reasonable hope of cure by the performance of an operation for evacuating its contents, is much smaller than most persons are aware of. There are two conditions or circumstances which preclude the probability—it may almost be said, the possibility—of the operation proving successful. 1. The existence of a plurality of abscesses. 2. An ulcerated state of the large intestines, or in other words, the co-existence of dysentery. Let us see in how many of the 300 fatal cases, given in the first part of this paper, the operation under these circumstances would have been applicable.

Total number of cases	300
There were a plurality of abscesses in ...	108
	192
Of the 177 cases in which the abscess was solitary, there was more or less extensive ulceration of the large intestines in	76
	116

Thus it appears, that out of the whole number, only in 116, or little more than 1 in 3, could the operation have been undertaken with any reasonable probability of success; and this number would, of course, be still further diminished, by taking into consideration the cases in which the abscess, though solitary, communicated with the lung, colon, or some other viscera, and those in which other organic disease existed.

Important, as it must be admitted, statistical data, such as the above are, in all disease, yet too much reliance should not be placed upon them when the question actually presents itself, whether or no an operation should be undertaken in any individual case. Under such circumstances, the surgeon must rely on his own judgment as to the propriety of undertaking it; the condition of the patient, his strength of constitution, the extent of the disease, the complication with other lesions, &c., all these should have the first consideration.

The exploratory needle mentioned as having been used with the trocar in 19 cases,(a) was first brought prominently to the notice of Indian medical officers by the late Drs. Mouat and Murray, in 1839. The principle acted upon was, that the sooner the contents of the abscess were evacuated, the greater was the chance of the patient's recovery; that if the operation were delayed until the disease had far advanced, until fluctuation became evident, and until the constitution became impaired, as evidenced by hepatic fever, cold sweats, &c., the chances of recovery were greatly diminished; and that the chief cause of the repeated failure of the operation was the delaying it, until, by these signs, the existence of hepatic abscess was placed beyond a doubt. A somewhat similar view of the question is expressed by the late Mr. Twining. (*Diseases of Bengal, 2d Ed.*, vol. i, *p.* 302.) In order to ascertain then, at an early period, the existence (or not) of abscess in the liver, they proposed and practised the mode of introducing an exploratory needle into the viscus. They doubtless held in view, when first proposing this bold line of practice, the fact, that the spleen, a much more vascular organ than the liver, may be punctured with perfect safety.(b) The needle employed in these cases was 3 or 4 inches long, with a canal in its centre in place of the groove—an important improvement on the old instrument.

As I find this treatment has been strongly condemned by a recent writer, (Mr. M. Stovell, *Trans. of the Med. and Phys. Society of Bombay*, No. 1, N. S., *p.* 188,) I shall adduce a few cases, in addition to the histories given previously,(a) as illustrative of the safety, if not of the success of this mode of treatment;—

(*a*) Cases v, vi, viii, xxi, xxii, xxiii, xxiv, xxv, xxvi, xxxiii, xxxv, xxxix, xli, xlvii, xlviii, l. li, lii, lv.

(*b*) See Twining, op. cit, vol. i, p. 450. Dr. G. Smith, Madras Med. Reports, 1850, p. 97.

but it does not appear from the data which I have been able to collect, that the practice is more successful, than when the trocar alone is employed.

Summary of Cases in which the Liver was explored without the evacuation of the contents of the abscess.

First Case. Recovered.—D. Derrick, H. M. 4th Regt., admitted Aug., 1839. On the 11th, the exploratory needle was introduced posteriorly to the angle of, and between the 7th and 8th ribs, to the depth of 2½ inches, but without detecting pus. No inconvenience ensued from the puncture, and the second day after the operation, the abscess apparently burst into the intestines, and he gradually recovered from that date. *He never experienced any bad symptoms from the introduction of the needle;* he thinks, on the contrary, that it rather did him good. *(Dr. Mouat, Madras Med. Journal,* vol. ii, *p.* 226.)

Second Case. Fatal.—J. Austen, H. M. 4th Regt.—detailed history not given—liver explored in two places without finding matter. On dissection, it was found that he had abscesses in both lobes. *The puncture with the exploratory needle had healed, without producing any bad effects. (Dr. Mouat, ibid, p.* 227.)

Third Case. Recovered.—A. Killagher, H. M. 39th Regt.—operated on July 22d, 1839—trocar only employed—pushed in its full length—blood only escaped—no pus—afforded great relief—canula left in the wound, with the view of preventing the escape of blood into the peritoneal cavity, and exciting adhesion between the liver and side—it was removed the following night, as it gave much pain. The prognosis was most unfavourable previous to the operation, after which however he gradually improved. Invalided, and sent to England. *(Dr. J. McGrigor, ibid,* vol. ii, *p.* 227.)

Fourth Case. Fatal.—H. McEvoy, H. M. 4th Regt., æt. 35, admitted April 28th, 1840—operated on May 28th—exploratory needle passed twice on different occasions into the liver, without detecting pus; the operation gave very little pain at the time—no subsequent uneasiness, and the puncture healed without any bad effect. He died Aug. 17th, 20 days after the operation.

Autopsy.—Liver adhering to contiguous viscera—several abscesses in both lobes—one had discharged its contents into the thoracic cavity. See further No. 30 in List of Cases. *(Dr. Allman, Madras Med. Journ.,* vol. iii, *p.* 193.)

Fifth Case. Fatal.—M. Sheard, H. M. 15th Hussars, admitted Nov. 22d, 1841—operated on Dec. 12th—exploratory needle introduced in two places, first at the epigastrium close to the edge of the false ribs, and secondly, through the intercostal muscles at the sternal extremity of the 9th and 10th ribs, but no purulent matter was detected. Died Jan. 6th, 26 days after the operation. Complicated with dysentery.

Autopsy.—Serous effusion into abdominal cavity—abscesses in both lobes of the liver, the cicatrices of the punctures were distinctly seen on the surface of the liver; neither of them had reached an abscess. One puncture entering the thorax in contact with a serration of the diaphragm, had passed through that muscle and penetrated the viscus, giving rise to effusion of lymph, with adhesions between the opposed surfaces of the serous membrane. Colon ulcerated. See further No. 45 in List of Cases. *(Dr. Mouat, ibid,* vol. iv, *p.* 187.)

Sixth Case. Fatal.—J. Spurway, H. M. 4th Regt., admitted May 14th, 1840. The exploratory needle was introduced at three different points into the liver without detecting pus. "These explorations occasioned scarcely any uneasiness to the patient at the time, and were unattended by the slightest ill consequence." He died on the 40th day after admission, and on dissection, it was found that he had several abscesses in the liver all beyond the reach of the needle. No. 56 in List of Cases. *(Dr. Parry, ibid,* vol. v, *p.* 321.)

These cases tend to show that the mere fact of exploring the liver is unattended with imminent danger or any immediate ill consequence.

Best period for the operation. It is of much practical importance to ascertain, if possible, whether a greater measure of success attends those cases in which the abscess is evacuated at an early period, than those in which the operation is delayed until the constitutional symptoms, unequivocally establish the fact of its existence. That the evacuation of these abscesses at an early period is desirable and advantageous, is an opinion I entertain, in common, I believe, with most of my medical brethren in India. It is however extremely difficult to obtain sufficient data whereon to base an opinion with any degree of certainty.

Below is given a table shewing the number of days the patients were in hospital before the operation was performed, together with the results of the same, at each period—but any deductions drawn from it, as to the advantage of early evacuation, must be received with great caution, as it is impossible to say to what extent the abscess may have progressed previous to admission; in some, the formation of the abscess may have commenced at some date subsequent to admission, whilst in others, the disease may have progressed to a great extent and fluctuation may have been evident, at the very period when the patients first applied for treatment.

Table shewing the number of days each patient was in hospital, previous to the abscess being evacuated.

	Number.	Recoveries	Deaths	Per centage of recoveries.
Under 10 days	8	3	5	35.500
From 10 to 20	14	2	12	14.285
„ 20 to 30	14	2	12	14.285
„ 30 to 40	3	0	3	——
„ 40 to 50	3	1	2	33.333
„ 50 to 100	9	3	6	33.333
Above 100 days	2	0	2	——
Not stated	28	4	24	14.286
	81	15	66	18.519

From this it appears, that although a larger proportion of recoveries took place when the operation was performed at an early period, especially under the first ten days, yet that a success, very little inferior to this, attended those cases in which the operation has been delayed for a long period. As before observed, however, this table, and consequently any deductions from it, are to be received with caution. No less necessary is this same caution if we turn to the fact of fluctuation being present, or not—the fact of there being fluctuation is of little value, unless we know whether the operation was undertaken immediately after it was first detected, or whether it was delayed for weeks perhaps after it was first noticed. We give the figures however as they stand.

	Number.	Recoveries	Deaths	Per centage of recoveries.
Fluctuation evident. .	27	9	18	33.333
No fluctuation present	5	1	4	20.000
	32	10	22	

If we may draw any deduction from these figures, it is that greater success attends those cases in which fluctuation was perceptible before the operation was commenced. The fact of fluctuation being present or absent, is not noticed in 49 cases.

This portion of the enquiry, a highly important one, is very imperfect; we much want good data whereon to base a sound estimate of the period which is best suited for the evacuation of these abscesses. This must be left to future enquirers—my own impression is, that the most eligible period for opening hepatic abscesses, is within a very short time, a few days, after fluctuation is perceptible—fluctuation once evident, the sooner the operation is performed the better.

Pus had escaped into the abdominal cavity in two cases, (xix, lxxviii,) in one of these the lancet had been employed, in the other the instrument used is not specified. It appears that the danger attending upon puncturing abscesses before adhesions are established, has been somewhat exaggerated—witness case iii, where, although the patient lived fourteen days after the operation, it was found on dissection, that no adhesion to the side had taken place, and yet not a drop of pus had escaped into the abdominal cavity. The danger, however, is not an imaginary one, as we see that this accident did occur in two cases in the above limited number. In the preceding cases, adhesion between the liver and side was found, on dissection, to be present in 31 cases, absent in two, (iii, xix,) and partial in one, (lxxviii.) Amongst the first class, the adhesions had doubtless in many cases existed before the operation was performed; but in others it was evident that these had taken place subsequently. In case vii, it is expressly stated that previous to the operation, there was no adhesion between the liver and the abdominal parietes; this man died of some other disease, six months after, and it was then found that there were no adhesions to any part of the side, except at the point where the puncture had been made, and at this spot it appeared as if it were attached to the walls of the abdomen, or rather hung from it by a cord about the size of a small goose quill. Case xxxiii and xxxiv, are also examples of the same fact; in both of these, the opening made by the trocar had become converted into a sort of canal formed by effused coagulable lymph. In these cases the trocar was used, and the canula left in situ. The reader may also refer to No. 64 in list of Fatal Cases, and case lxviii in the list of operations, for the description of the adhesions in persons who survived the operation some years.

The very early period at which these adhesions begin to form, is alike interesting and important. In case xvi, the patient died the day after the operation was performed, and in case v, two days after; in both these, adhesions were found to be commencing, some lymph being effused in each around the site of the puncture—the trocar was the instrument used in both these cases.

It would be highly presumptive in me, with my limited experience, to pass a decided opinion as to the best instrument for the purpose of evacuating these abscesses; but, from the perusal of a large number of cases, and from some little practical observation, it appears to me that the trocar is the best adapted for the purpose, especially as the canula, if left in the puncture, not only prevents the escape of matter should the liver collapse, or shrink after the operation, but its presence tends, by creating some little irritation, to cause the more rapid effusion of coagulable lymph, and thus the more readily to establish adhesions at this point. A flat trocar, as recommended by the late Dr. Murray, Inspector-General, may be preferable to the common round one in some cases.

The mode of ascertaining if adhesions exist. The importance of ascertaining whether adhesions exist between the liver and the abdominal parietes, previous to undertaking the operation for the evacuation of the contents of an hepatic abscess, is very evident; although, as before observed, perhaps the importance attached to it, has been somewhat exaggerated. The stethoscope, in such cases, affords us valuable information. The peritoneal friction sound, or "Leather creak," was first shown by Dr. Bright,(a) (*Med. Chir. Trans.*, vol. xix, *p.* 177, *et seq.*) to be diagnostic of adhesion having taken place between the liver and the abdominal parietes; and in four cases which are given by way of illustration, dissection proved the diagnosis to have been correct. Dr. Corrigan, however, (*Dublin Journ. of Med. Sciences*, July, 1836,) has adduced a case in which this sound was heard, and after death, it was found that adhesion had not taken place, but there was found a layer of moderately firm rough spongy lymph, with small tubercles, between the opposing surfaces of the peritoneum. Piorry, (*Traité de la Percussion, p.* 159,) considers this sound as diagnostic of the presence of hydatids; but, as in none of the cases adduced by Drs. Bright or Corrigan, any hydatids were present, we are justified in rejecting this hypothesis. I believe that I am correct, in stating, that the best English authorities agree in the opinion of Dr. Bright, that this sound is diagnostic of adhesion having taken place. Thus we find that Professor Walshe, in an excellent lecture on a case of hepatic abscess, says, "this objection (want of adhesion to the parietes) did not hold here, because I discovered distinct peritoneal friction sound over the prominence—*the clear*

(*a*) Is this correct? Was not this sound first discovered by Mr. Malcolmson? I have not Mr. M.'s paper in No. liii, of the Edin. Med. and Surg. Journal, to refer to.

proof that local adhesive inflammation had arisen in the desired loca''.y." (*Lancet*, 1849, vol. ii, *p.* 525.)

This sound is described by Dr. Bright, as "a very peculiar sensation communicated to the touch, varying between the crepitation produced by emphysema, and the sensation of bending new leather in the hand; or that experienced when the finger or hand is rubbed over a damp pane of glass." Piorry speaks of it, as "a mixed sensation perceived at the same instant by the ear and finger." Dr. Corrigan says, that it is easily recognized, although with difficulty described. "We are conscious," he observes, "when we squeeze or bend new leather so as to make it creak, that we receive a peculiar sensation simultaneously through the ear and finger,—a sensation as if the impression on the hearing were conveyed through the finger touching the leather. Such is this sign as near as I can describe it. In cases where the creaking may be indistinct to the sense of touch, the stethoscope is of great assistance in detecting it. The instrument is to be applied over the part of the abdomen where the creak is sought for, while at the same time the parietes of the abdomen are pressed with a moderate degree of firmness and suddenness with the hand; the creaking will be heard loud by the ear while it is dull to the finger." This sound very closely resembles the "Bruit de Cuir Neuf," observed in pericarditis, but it is more prolonged, louder, and coarser.

The mechanism of this sound is a matter of doubt. Dr. Bright, as we have seen, attributes it to the existence of adhesions; Recamier and Piorry to the presence of hydatids, and Dr. Beatty, (*Dublin Med. Journal*, vol. vi,) to the rubbing together of the opposing surfaces of the peritoneum which have become rough from the deposition of lymph. This last opinion is also entertained by Dr. Corrigan, to whose able paper on this subject the reader is referred for more full details.

SUMMARY

OF

TWENTY-FIVE CASES OF HEPATIC ABSCESS

WHICH TERMINATED IN SPONTANEOUS RECOVERY.

Case 1. *Opening into the abdominal cavity* (?)—Grogan, had a long protracted convalescence from fever, followed in the first instance by fixed acute pain in the epigastrium, with enlargement of the liver, and vomiting; and afterwards by a sensation of something giving way or bursting, subsidence of the swelling, general severe abdominal pain, and collapse. No pus was evacuated by vomiting nor by stool, yet he recovered and was reported "well" some months after. *(Dr. J. Murray, Madras Medical Journal,* vol. i, *p.* 80.)

Case 2. *Opening into the colon.*—The particulars of this case not given. It is merely stated that the abscess burst into the colon; the puriform discharge persisted for 20 days, and the patient convalesced rapidly. *(Dr. J. Murray, ibid, p.* 80.*)*

Case 3. *Pus passed in the urine.*—W. Gettings, æt. 26, 6 years in India; admitted with hepatitis, Jan. 7th, 1838. The symptoms were well marked—copious ptyalism established early—had rigors, cold sweats, pain in the side and shoulder, &c.—a seton inserted in the side. On the 30th day after admission, he commenced passing purulent matter in his urine—this discharge continued for seven days and nights, and after this was no longer visible, the urine became clear and copious, and his health became daily better. He was discharged convalescent, March 18th, 40 days after the purulent matter was first observed in the urine—active counter-irritation by setons, blisters, &c. was kept up in this case. *(Dr. J. P. Grant, ibid,* vol. i, *p.* 326.*)*

Case 4. *Spontaneous absorption?*—Corporal Quins, H. M. 80th Regt. This man had apparently a very large abscess—the tumour was very large at the epigastrium, but it had a flat indolent appearance without any distinct margin, although *fluctuation was pretty distinct.* He was put on nourishing diet—took Pulv.

Digitatis in doses, grains 1 and 2 hourly—a plaster was put round the ribs to support the parts, and he was given nitrous acid internally. He gradually recovered, and at the period of the report was described as "in robust health." State of the urine, stools, &c., not given. *(Dr. Nicoll, Madras Medical Journal,* vol. iii, *p.* 269.)

Case 5. *Pus passed in the urine.*—W. Harrier, æt. 25, admitted with acute hepatitis, Dec. 3d, 1841—the symptoms severe, the treatment active, ptyalism established on the 6th day. There was much fulness of the side, pain increased by pressure, cold sweats, &c.—percussion elicited a dull sound from the 6th rib downwards. On the 13th, he was seized with acute pain in the region of the left kidney, occasionally shooting across the abdomen—he had also some slight *ardor urinæ,* the ptyalism continued unabated. On the 20th, (17 days after admission,) his urine, which had hitherto been quite clear, contained about two ounces of a thick white deposit; this, which closely resembled pus, continued for eight days, and in the mean time, all the prominent symptoms, the swelling of the side, the pain on pressure, the rigors, &c., gradually subsided; and the last report is, "No complaint with the exception of debility." The purulent sediment in the urine continued till the 28th, and the urine itself had a strong ammoniacal odour. *(Dr. C. D. Currie, Madras Med. Journal,* vol. iv, *p.* 385.)

Case 6. *Spontaneous absorption?*—M. Thompson, H. M. 4th Regt. A large tumour formed to the right of the ensiform cartilage, in which obscure fluctuation was detected, which was preceded by rigors, and accompanied with hectic. The case was seen by several experienced medical officers, and abscess was positively diagnosed, but while the propriety of puncturing the tumour was under consideration, it disappeared, and the man got perfectly well. He afterwards improved much in flesh and strength, although an old worn out debauchee. *(Dr. F. W. Innes, Madras Medical Journal,* vol. vi, *p.* 175.)

Case 7. *Opening into the intestines.*—Particulars not given. It is simply stated that the abscess burst into the intestines, and the contents were passed by stool. The man at the date of the report was perfectly convalescent. *(Dr. Innis, ibid, p.* 176.*)*

Case 8. *Opening into the abdominal cavity?*—E. A., æt. 37, admitted with hepatitis, for which he was leeched and took calomel till the gums were affected. A tumour now presented itself in the right hypochondrium, and there was considerable swelling with hardness of the side—he was much troubled with flatulence and spasms. On the 13th day of treatment he had severe spasms, attended by profuse perspiration, which in the arms and hands was cold and clammy; the pulse rose to 120; countenance sunken; voice weak. On examining the side, the swelling had in a great measure subsided, but there was fulness in the lower part of the abdomen, and he could lie in positions that formerly gave him pain. He passed no pus by stool, nor is any mention made of his passing any in the urine, or by vomiting. The report only continues for a short time after this date, but he was apparently convalescing. He afterwards embarked for England. (*Dr. C. J. Cowie, ibid*, vol. vi, *p.* 176.)

Case 9. *Opening into the abdominal cavity?*—This case is very similar to the last, only not so well marked. P. F., æt. 21, admitted Oct. 21st, 1835, with hepatitis, for which he was bled locally and generally, and he took mercury till his mouth was sore, although it does not appear that healthy ptyalism was established. There was distinct enlargement with hardness of the left lobe of the liver. On December 2d, he was seized with severe pain suddenly in the abdomen, and vomited a good deal; at the same time, the swelling in the epigastric region decreased, and the lower part of the abdomen became distended. He had much abdominal uneasiness for some time, but from this date, improvement commenced, and at the date of the last report, he was convalescent. (*Dr. R. Davidson, ibid*, vol. vi, *p.* 184.)

Case 10. *Opening into the colon.*—J. Millwood, æt. 22, admitted with hepatitis, Dec. 20th, 1812—was purged, &c., and took mercury, but not to the extent of affecting the system. On the 19th of January, (30 days after admission,) he felt something break immediately under the umbilicus, and discharged per anum a quantity of thick matter like cream; he felt immediate ease—much flatus—belly tense. This discharge continued with some variation as to its consistence, &c. for 17 days. He was discharged, Feb. 12th, (24 days after the presumed bursting of the abscess,) and was in good health four years afterwards. (*Annesley, Diseases of India, 4to Ed.*, vol. i, *p.* 669.)

Case 11. *Opening into the colon.*—A. Murray, æt. 26, admitted with hepatitis, Jan. 7th, 1813. He was bled locally and generally, took calomel, purgatives, &c. On the 5th day of treatment, he had a sensation at night as if something had broken internally, and he had a very copious discharge per anum. On the 18th, the discharge had ceased, and a few days after he left hospital. Was in good health many years after. (*Annesley, ibid, p.* 671.)

Case 12. *Opening into the lungs.*—O. Keating, æt. 29, admitted July 3d, 1819, with dysenteric symptoms and hepatitis. On the 10th day, he was seized with a violent pain in the region of the liver, and cough with a sudden and great expectoration of pus. The quantity of pus expectorated in the first three hours amounted altogether to 3 pounds—breathing impeded—pain in the right side, chest, &c. On the 17th of July, a wound which he had received in his thigh, broke out and discharged a quantity of pus, with several small stones—this discharge continued for some days—that from the lungs ceased nine days after its commencement. For some time, he had much dyspnæa, with a short cough, &c.; he then gradually improved, and finally recovered perfectly. (*Annesley, ibid, p.* 673.)

Case 13. *Opening into the colon.*—A. Brapson, æt. 22, admitted with hepatitis, Nov. 9th, 1816—he was freely bled, leeched, &c., and took mercury till his mouth was sore—the symptoms of hepatic abscess well marked. On the 26th day of treatment, much matter was passed by stool, and it became evident that the abscess had burst into the intestines. In addition to pus, he passed blood in his stools, and this continued more or less for 37 days. From the time of its cessation, Dec. 14th, he gradually improved, and at last perfectly recovered. (*Annesley, ibid, Appendix, p.* xxxviii.)

Case 14. *Opening into the colon.*—J. M., æt. 42, admitted Oct. 19th, 1830, with hepatic derangement, purging, &c.; he was actively treated, bled locally and generally—had purgatives, and took calomel till his mouth was sore. On the 4th day after admission, there being at the time great evident enlargement of the liver, he passed above 1 pound of pus mixed with some florid blood, and at the same time, the swelling in the right hypochondrium decreased—he became very weak—had hectic, &c. The discharge continued for 17 days—the patient then gradually recovered, and became quite well. (*Twining, Diseases of Bengal,* vol. i, *p.* 307.)

Case 15. *Opening into the colon.*—J. Goddard, æt. 18, admitted Oct. 21st, 1827, with enlarged liver, pain in the shoulder, &c.; the cartilages of the false ribs were much elevated, and abscess in the liver was clearly diagnosed. On the 26th day after admission, he awoke with a great sense of faintness and nausea, and a frequent desire to go to stool, and he passed per anum about 1½ pound of pus and blood; the tumour at the side and epigastrium at the same time subsided considerably. The discharge continued for 11 days; he then very much improved and shortly after embarked for England. (*Twining, ibid,* vol. i, *p.* 307.)

Case 16. *Opening into the lungs.*— ——, æt. 34, under treatment for dyspepsia. On the 18th day of treatment, a troublesome cough came on, and on the 25th day, after the pain in the right side had commenced, a slight degree of bloody expectoration appeared. On the 26th day, he suddenly experienced a sense of suffocation and extreme faintness, and coughed up about 4½ ounces of thick, viscid, puriform matter. Hectic symptoms came on, and he became very low and weak, but the pain in the right side ceased. He went to sea, and gradually recovered his health. (*Twining, ibid*, vol. i, *p*. 342.)

Case 17. *Opening into the lungs.*—Lieut. R., æt. 51, subject to hepatic disease, admitted June 23d, 1842, with uneasiness in the right side, irregular bowels, loss of appetite, &c. On the 11th day of treatment, he was seized with a fit of coughing, and ejected about 6 ounces of frothy puriform fluid. This continued for 6 weeks, the quantity daily being sometimes several ounces; at times it was of a brick-red colour; it ceased on Aug. 17th; he left hospital, Sept. 6th, and proceeded to England, where he died shortly after, but under what circumstances is not known. (*Dr. Morehead, Trans. of the Med. and Phys. Society of Bombay*, vol. vii, *p*. 50.)

Case 18. *Opening into the lungs.*—E. Simmons, æt. 32, in India 2 years, admitted April 26th, 1847, with acute hepatitis, pain in side and shoulder, painful decubitus on the left side, &c. The symptoms, which were well marked, yielded to bleeding and purgatives, and to mercury carried to salivation. On May 12th, (20 days after the first symptoms,) he was suddenly seized with severe cough, and expectorated about 1½ pounds of pus; the pulse rose to 100, but he had no pain. On the following day, he expectorated a considerable quantity of pus, but it soon became less and less, and finally ceased by the 17th. He left the hospital quite well, June 8th, 27 days after the expectoration commenced.

Note.—Some years after, (1853) this man died of delirium tremens, having had no hepatic or pulmonary affection in the interval. The lower surface of the right lung, to the extent of about 3 inches, was closely adherent to the diaphragm, and there was a co-extensive adhesion between the diaphragm and the upper surface of the liver. The liver itself was slightly enlarged, yellowish, fatty, and friable. The lower portion of the right lung was hepatized to a slight extent. (*Mr. Stovell, Trans. of the Med. and Phys. Society of Bombay*, No. i, N. S., *p*. 168.)

Case 19. *Opening into the lungs.*—C. Steel, æt. 24, in India 3 months, admitted Nov. 18th, 1848, with acute hepatitis, having been ill three days. The symptoms were well marked, and partially yielded to bleeding, purgatives, &c.; he also took mercury till his mouth was affected. The pain subsided, but he had uneasiness in the side till Dec. 11th, (24 days after the first symptom,) when he suddenly expectorated 4 ounces of pus. For some days he continued to expectorate 6 or 8 ounces of thick, reddish pus. By the end of the month, this discharge totally ceased; his bowels, however, remained irritable for a time, but he gradually recovered strength, and left hospital, quite well, March 7th, 86 days after the expectoration commenced. *(Stovell, ibid, p.* 169.)

Case 20. *Opening into the lungs.*—R. Ramford, æt. 34, admitted Dec. 17th, 1849, with acute hepatitis, for which he was depleted, and took mercury until his gums were slightly tender. On the 25th, he was troubled with cough, and expectorated a small quantity of pus, which he felt distinctly coming from the side affected. This expectoration continued until Jan. 2d, and he was discharged quite well, 34 days after the abscess burst into the lungs. *(Stovell, ibid, p.* 171.)

Case 21. *Opening into the lungs.*—E. Miller, æt. 29, admitted April 24th, 1850, with hepatitis, of which he had been ill since March 10th. He had been freely depleted, and brought under the influence of mercury; he had still some pain under the margin of the right ribs, increased on pressure—bowels relaxed and irritable. On the 26th, (47 days from the first symptom,) he expectorated about an ounce of pus, mixed with blood and mucus; he continued to expectorate about two ounces daily till the end of the month. He remained weak, but left the hospital, May 14th, 19 days after the first expectoration of pus. *(Stovell, ibid, p.* 172.)

Case 22. *Opening into the lungs.*—E. Bevan, æt. 36, was under treatment for hepatitis from March 19th to April 8th, 1851. He was re-admitted, April 26th, having been drinking freely. On admission, he had just been seized with severe pain in the region of the liver, with cough and dyspnæa, and he was freely expectorating purulent matter, an abscess having evidently opened into the bronchi. This was 38 days from the date of first admission. For some days, the cough returned in paroxysms, lasting about an hour, and during each of these, he expectorated pus profusely, mixed with blood. On the 9th of May, the discharge ceased, and he left hospital well, June 2d, 37 days after the first purulent expectoration. *(Stovell, ibid, p.* 172.)

Case 23. *Opening into the lungs.*—G. Bulline, æt. 27, admitted Jan. 12th, 1852, with hepatitis, of which he had suffered several previous attacks. He was leeched, &c., and took mercury till it affected his gums, when all the urgent symptoms subsided. He now began to sweat profusely at nights, the bowels became irritable, and there was hepatic dulness as high as the mamma. On Feb. 2d, (21 days after admission,) he was awoke from his sleep by severe cough, and he expectorated 8 ounces of pus, an abscess having evidently opened into the bronchi. For some time, he continued to expectorate about 8 ounces of pus in the 24 hours, but chiefly at nights; he however improved in health, and the discharge gradually diminished till the end of March, when it finally ceased. He was discharged quite well, April 26th, 83 days after the first purulent expectoration. (*Stovell, ibid, p.* 173.)

Case 24. *Opening into the lungs.*—D. O'Connell, æt. 39, for years subject to hepatic derangement, admitted April 12th, 1852, with well marked hepatitis; there was also some fulness of the side, and hepatic dulness as high as the 4th rib. He was depleted, and took calomel till he began to sweat profusely at nights, when it was omitted. On the 23d, (11 days after admission,) he was seized with sudden dyspnæa and cough, and expectorated about 4 ounces of pus, an abscess having evidently opened into the bronchi. A similar amount of expectoration continued for some days; it then diminished, and by the beginning of May, it had entirely ceased. The night sweats disappeared, as well as all the other bad symptoms, and he was discharged well, May 24th, 32 days after the first purulent expectoration. (*Stovell, ibid, p.* 174.)

Case 25. *Two abscesses, one opening into the colon and another into the lungs.*—Mr. J. C. S., was attacked on Aug. 6th, 1836, with acute hepatitis, for which he was actively treated; the urgent symptoms subsided, but it soon became evident that abscess in the liver had formed. The treatment was now simply palliative. On the 13th of Sept., he was sensible of something having given way within him, and he all at once felt himself relieved of the distressing symptoms from which he had been suffering—a considerable quantity of purulent matter was found in the stools, and this was observed for several days subsequently. It was evident that the abscess had burst into the colon. At the end of 10 or 12 days, he became worse again, and all his old symptoms returned; slight hopes were entertained of his recovery. On the 4th of Oct. however, a change for the better commenced, and a large quantity of matter was discharged by expectoration; an abscess in the liver had evidently burst into the lungs. From this date, he continued to get better, and 6 weeks afterwards, (Nov. 22d,) the patient is reported as recovering rapidly. (*Dr. T. B. Colledge, in Webb's Pathologia Indica, p.* 296.)

REMARKS

ON

THE CASES OF HEPATIC ABSCESS

WHICH TERMINATED IN RECOVERY.

Recovery in 25 Cases took place:—

By the abscess opening into the lung, and the matter being discharged, by expectoration, through the bronchi[a] ...	10
By the abscess opening into the colon or some part of the large intestine, the contents being voided by stool[b] ...	7
By one abscess opening into the lungs, and another into the colon (Case 25.)	1
By the abscess discharging its contents into the abdominal cavity (?) (Cases 1, 8, 9.)	3
By the elimination of pus by the kidney (Cases 3, 5.) ...	2
By spontaneous absorption (?) (Cases 4, 6.)...	2
	25

Of the first two modes of recovery, there is little to observe, except that it appears, (if indeed we are entitled to draw any conclusion from such limited data,) that the most favourable position for an hepatic abscess to open, is into the lung;—at any rate, we are justified in saying, as far as these cases are concerned, that the largest proportion recovered, when the abscess opened in this site.

With respect to those abscesses which are described as opening into the abdominal cavity, I think that the diagnosis should be received with caution; it seems almost incredible that pus in any quantity should come in contact with a serous membrane, so exquisitely sensitive as the peritoneum, without giving rise to such an amount of inflammation as would almost certainly prove fatal; and it does not appear from the two cases in which the histories are fully detailed, (8 and 9,) that any notable amount of peritonitis followed the symptoms which were supposed to indicate the burst-

(a) Cases 12, 16, 17, 18, 19, 20, 21, 22, 23, 24.
(b) Cases 2, 7, 10, 11, 13, 14, 15.

ing of the abscess into the abdominal cavity. If the reader will turn to No. 64, in the List of Fatal Cases, and will compare the symptoms therein detailed, with those given in the two others now under consideration, he will find a very strong similarity in all the principal features. In the fatal case, there was the same sudden accession of pain, with collapse, cold sweats, sunken countenance, rapid pulse, &c., and without any attendant purulent discharge, either by stool, urine or expectoration, yet dissection showed that no pus had escaped into the peritoneal cavity, and that the intestines and abdominal viscera were healthy. The reporter of this case, (Dr. Pollock,) himself confesses that he is quite at a loss to account for the symptoms which appeared to him, clearly to indicate the rupture of the abscess into the abdominal cavity.

No. 35, in the Fatal Cases, is highly interesting, as shewing the manner in which recovery might *possibly* take place even after the abscess had actually burst into this cavity; here the escaped matter had given rise to inflammation, and the adhesions formed by the effused lymph, had confined the purulent matter in a separate sac. The case is well worthy of the attention of the reader.

The cases which are described as cured by the elimination of pus by the kidneys, are fraught with much interest and importance, in no small degree increased by the mystery in which the subject is involved. Here we have two cases in which the appearance of a white sediment (considered by competent authority to have been purulent matter) in the urine, was followed by the immediate improvement and the subsequent recovery of the patient. If we turn to the histories of the Fatal Cases, we find six (No. 13, 30, 45, 223, 224, 227,) in which the urine was purulent, and yet dissection could detect no communication between the hepatic abscess and the kidneys, or any other portion of the urinary organs; in like manner, purulent matter was observed in the stools in several instances, (17, 30, 32, 41, 58, 148, 271,) and yet in none did the abscess apparently communicate with any part of the intestinal canal.

How are these facts to be explained? The much larger diameter of the pus corpuscule compared with the calibre of the capillary vessels, has been regarded by many physiologists, Muller, Budd, &c., as conclusive of the impossibility of the purulent contents of these abscesses being removed or carried into the circulation, and subsequently eliminated by the blood vessels. This objection, though a very powerful one, is not insurmountable, as we know that under certain circumstances, the capillaries may be dilated to such an extent as to permit bodies of even larger (comparative) dimensions than the pus corpuscule to pass through them. However difficult it may be to reconcile this theory with physiological facts, it is the only explanation, that I am aware of, which will satisfactorily explain in any degree, the various phenomena detailed in connexion with this subject; besides which, we have some sort of proof, not conclusive, it must be admitted, that this explanation is the true one. Thus Twining states, (*Diseases of Bengal*, vol. i, *p.* 232,) that on two occasions, in persons who had died of hepatic abscess, he found a small quantity of puriform matter in the right ventricle of the heart, and in both instances, he was able to trace the same appearance, with small filamentous coagula, back through the auricle, and along the vena cava, quite into the veins of the liver. Mühlbauer also relates a case of a man who had several abscesses in the lungs and about his body; on examining his body after death, there was found in the cavities of the heart, a small quantity of thin fluid blood, having a dirty brownish appearance; under the microscope, there were discovered, besides blood corpuscules, a considerable quantity of large granulated corpuscules presenting all the characters of ordinary pus corpuscules, and, like these, rendered transparent by treatment with acetic acid, whereupon a cup-shaped nucleus in each was brought into view. (*Schmidt's Jahrbücher*, Heft. ii, 1845.)

Again, Prof. Walshe, in his Clinical Lecture on Hepatic Abscess, more than once alluded to before, speaking of the urine in a case he had under treatment, states that it was albuminous, and at one time contained corpuscules of a peculiar character; these were a third larger than blood discs, granulated, spherical, and disclosed a distinct nucleus under the action of acetic acid; some of them were isolated, others aggregated and associated with epithelium scales in great abundance, having the character of those of muco-pus. (*Lancet*, 1849, vol. ii, *p.* 525.)

Lastly, in three cases observed by Dr. Conwell, (No. 216, 218, 220 in the Fatal Cases,) pus was detected in the kidneys themselves, although no connexion between these organs and the abscess could be discovered.

I do not see how these facts can be explained, excepting by the supposition that the purulent contents of the abscess were absorbed by the hepatic vessels, were thus carried into the circulation, and subsequently eliminated by the blood vessels.

Dr. Mouat has published a list of 13 cases of hepatic abscess, in which the purulent contents were apparently thrown off in a vicarious manner. I regret that I have not the volume (3d) of the *Quart. Journal of the Calcutta Med. and Phys. Society*, to refer to for the particulars. In the *Madras Journal*, vol. ii, *p.* 20, the same authority gives a table of 109 patients who passed purulent matter by urine, 33 of the number also by stool, and 8 of them *pus* by expectoration; but it does not appear that all these were cases of hepatic abscesses.

Dr. Budd, (op. cit. *p.* 89,) considers that these deposits regarded as purulent, are not so in reality, but that in all probability, they were simply a deposit of the phosphates. To aid future investigators, I shall take the liberty of quoting a passage from Dr. Garrod's Lectures on the Chemistry of Pathology. (*Lancet*, 1848, vol. ii, *p.* 625.)

"Urine containing pus," he observes, "is usually acid in its re-actions, and also albuminous, the albumen being derived from the liquor puris, which to a certain extent resembles the serum of the blood. The amount of albumen is generally small, and proportionate to the quantity of pus globules which are present; such urine has little tendency to become alkaline. Under the microscope, the pus globules are easily distinguished, consisting of cells larger than blood discs, of a whitish colour, and strongly granular on their surfaces. On the addition of acetic acid, several nuclei become visible. When purulent urine is allowed to stand for a little time, the globules subside and form a whitish deposit, not unlike some phosphatic sediments; and if it should become alkaline by putrefaction, and the generation of ammonia takes place, then the pus becomes altered in character, viscid, glairy and ropy, and with difficulty diffused through the fluid. The addition of acetic acid again restores the pus to its former state of a granular deposit. By these re-actions and appearances taken together, deposits of pus are distinguished from those consisting of mucus, either derived from the urinary passages, or from the presence of mucous discharge from the genital organs, as leucorrhœa, &c. These last, however, sometimes assume a purulent character."

With respect to the cases said to be cured by spontaneous absorption, much mystery exists as to the mode in which the cure is effected; it is not improbable that the puriform deposit may have been eliminated from the system in the secretions, and have escaped the observation of the medical attendant. No. 6, is peculiarly interesting; no doubt of there being an abscess could exist, and yet in how mysterious a manner did recovery ensue.

TREATMENT.

It was not originally my intention to have entered upon the subject of treatment of hepatic abscess, the enquiry being limited to the Pathology and Statistics of the affection, and with my very limited experience, it would savour strongly of presumption to offer any remarks of my own on the subject. I cannot, however, refrain from offering a few reflections which have occurred to me whilst penning the foregoing cases.

1. The most energetic treatment of an original affection, especially if it be of an active, inflammatory character, such as hepatitis or dysentery, affords no security against the supervention of suppurative inflammation of the liver. No. 33, 68, 69 and 70, may be consulted as illustrative of this proposition.

2. Mercury is a remedy of very doubtful utility; its free exhibition is undoubtedly no preventitive of hepatic abscess. Out of the 300 cases admitted under various headings, mercury was exhibited in one form or another in 135 cases: of this number it caused distinct salivation in 18, and in 17 others, it produced a sore or ulcerated state of the gums, but without free or proper ptyalism; in 19 others it appears to have been given with an unsparing hand, but without producing its specific effects on the system. It appears certain that the *early* establishment of salivation in hepatitis, dysentery, or fever, affords no security against the subsequent invasion of abscess in the liver, for we find that in two instances, (68, 69,) ptyalism was established within a few days after admission, and the mouth remained sore nearly up to the period of death; and in several others, (35, 70, 160, 183, 228,) mercury appears to have been given freely and early, before any evidence of the existence of hepatic abscess presented itself. In some cases[(a)] mercury seems to have been productive of more or less temporary benefit; in others (163,) it does not appear to have mitigated any of the symptoms, and in others (89,) it was obliged to be discontinued from the fact of its causing irritation. To aid those who are anxious to examine further the subject of mercury in these cases, there is added in the Appendix the numbers in the Fatal Cases, in which the action of mercury is noticed.

(a) Cases 3, 39, 45, 54, 55, 79, 126, 127, 131, 178.

I think that it may fairly be admitted as a question whether mercury, by its stimulant action on the secretory apparatus of the liver, does not act prejudicially in these cases, and whether it does not tend, by its stimulant property, to promote rather than retard the supervention of hepatic abscess. I am not in a position to state positively as a fact that this is so, nor am I prepared unhesitatingly to say that such is my belief, but I think, that a perusal of the preceding fatal cases, engenders and justifies a very strong suspicion, that mercury does tend, in conjunction with some other circumstances hitherto undetermined, to produce that condition of the liver which terminates in suppuration.

This is a subject of the deepest practical importance, and one to which the practitioner should pay the most serious attention, as the question of the beneficial or injurious action of mercury, in relation to hepatic abscess, can only be satisfactorily determined, by close and unremitting observation at the bed side of the patient. There can be no question as to its injurious action after suppuration has taken place.

3. The repeated use of strong purgatives tends much to debilitate the patient, and is attended with no commensurate benefit. The practitioner should be satisfied with an open or free state of the bowels, without giving medicines to produce violent purging, with the view of bringing away vitiated secretions, which probably do not exist. Many of the vitiated, green, watery stools, mentioned in these cases, are evidently the creation of the doctor himself—being produced by the purgatives which he has administered.

4. Whenever, in the course of an acute attack of hepatitis, or dysentery, or fever, occurring in India, symptoms indicative of hepatic abscess, appear—the persistence in all active or energetic measures, more especially the administration of mercury, seems to exercise an injurious influence—reducing the strength of the patient, without diminishing the local affection.

5. The remedies which under these circumstances seem to hold out the best prospect of success, are the various preparations of iodine, especially the iodide of potassium—the iodide of mercury may also prove serviceable in some instances—and the liquor arsenici et hydrargyri iodidi may be tried with advantage—the strong tincture of iodine being applied over the hepatic region at the same time. Mr. Twining's objections to the use of iodine in hepatic affections appear to have been founded on insufficient data. The above preparations of iodine may be advantageously combined with sedatives, especially with hyoscyamus or conium—opium appearing in some cases to interfere with the action of these salts.

Dilute nitric acid internally, at the same time that the nitro-muriatic acid lotion is applied externally, certainly appears to have in some cases, a most beneficial effect. Large, warm, soft, but not heavy poultices to the side, mild tonics, especially the citrate of iron and quinine, and a light nutritious diet, appear to be, amongst other measures, best adapted to the treatment of these cases. The use of all spirituous and vinous liquors, especially the more diffusible stimulants, requires great circumspection. Repeated relays of leeches to the side appear of questionable utility, tending rather to derive blood *to* the liver and *from* it; applied to the verge of the anus, however, they often appear to prove most beneficial in relieving hepatic congestions.

6. Counter-irritation, judiciously employed, is also a powerful agent for good; but the kind of agent must be suited to the case—in bronchial, or abdominal *irritation* or inflammation, without effusion, simple external irritants, as the tartar emetic ointment, prove most beneficial—in all serous effusions, those irritants properly denominated vesicants, are the most suitable in promoting absorption; but when the fluid to be absorbed is purulent, neither of these classes of irritants are of much benefit—then we must have recourse to setons and issues, and a free *purulent* discharge kept up. These are most valuable agents, but caution is necessary in their use; they are inadmissible whilst pyrexia exists. The quantity of the discharge should not be such as to weaken the patient more than can be helped.

Lastly, when all these measures fail in arresting the progress of the case, and fluctuation gives us decided evidence of the fact of abscess being present—the best prospect of success, is to evacuate the contents by operation.

BIBLIOGRAPHY.

The following list of works or articles having reference to hepatic abscess, is added in order to aid those who wish to investigate the subject in a more extended manner than is done in the preceding pages. It does not pretend to be a complete Bibliographical Record.

Hippocrates, *De Morbis*, Leyden, 1564, Lib. i, p. 150, and Lib. ii, p. 169.—Aretæus, in *Stephani's Med. Art. Principes*, 1567, Lib. i, p. 32.—Celsus in *ibid*, *Art. C. Celsus.*—Galen, *Method. Medendi Ed. Argentorati*, 1504, Lib. xiii.—Aëtius, *Zetrabib*, Lib. iii, Sect. ii.—Albucasis, *Ed. Oxon.*, 1778, Vol. i, p. 61.—Morgagni, *Epist.*, xxxvi, n. v.—Boerhaave, *Aphorisms by Van Swieten, Ed.* Edinburgh, 1776, Vol. ix, p. 208.—Bogue, in *Lind's Essay on Dis. of Hot Climates*, *2d Ed.*, London, 1771, p. 102, (abscess opened.)—T. Short, *Phil. Trans.*, 1731, Abr. vii, p. 500.—Sir E. Barry, *Edin. Med. Essays*, 1732, p. 273.—Dundas, *Edin. Med. Essays*, 1733, Vol. ii, p. 345.—Jamieson, *ibid*, Vol. iv., p. 425, 1745, (passed by stool.)—Sir W. Fordyce, *Fragmenta Chirurg. et Medica*, Lond. 1784.—Asper, in *Richter's Chirurg. Biblioth.*, Vol. iv, p. 765, 1777.—Haasius, *De Abscessibus Hepatis, Frank. Del. Op.*, 8vo, 1788.—J. Clark of Dominica, *Med. Commentaries* for 1789, Vol. xiv, p. 317, (13 abscesses opened.)—T. Garnett, *Med. Comment.* for 1788, Vol. xiii, p. 303, (passed by stool.)—Simmons, *Med. and Phys. Journal* for 1803, (abscess opened—recovery.)—Curtis, *Diseases of India*, Edin. 8vo, 1807, p. 100, *seq.*—Sir J. Pringle, *Obs. on the Diseases of the Army*, 1810, p. 146.—Sir J. McGrigor, in *Annals of Med.* for 1801, p. 363.—Saunders, *On the Liver*, 1803, p. 224.—Baron Larrey, *Mem. de Chirurg. Militaire*, Paris, 1812–17, Tom. ii, p. 51, 54.—Marshall, *Med. Topog. of Ceylon*, 1821, p. 150.—Portal, *Sur les Malad. du Foie*, Paris, 1813, and *Anat. Médicale*, t. v, p. 304.—Sir G. Ballingall, *Pract. Obs. on Fever, &c.* p. 102, 109.—Louis, *Sur les Abcés du Foie* in *Mem. on Recherch. Anat. Patholog.*, Paris, 1826.—Petit, *Mem. de l'Acad. de Chir.*, 12mo, Vol. i, p. 255, (abscess opened into colon after a second abscess had been evacuated by operation.)—Graves, *Dublin Med. Journal*, No. xiv, p. 349, (abscess opening into pericardium.)—Horner, *American Journal of Med. Sciences*, xiv, p. 87, 1834, (liver stitched to the side, there being no adhesions—death.)—Abercrombie, *Diseases of the Stomach, &c. 3d Ed.*, 1837, p. 320, (four cases.)—Malcolmson, *Edin. Med. Surg. Journal*, lii, p. 351, and in *Med. Chir. Trans.*, xxi, p. 19.—Stokes, *Art. Liver in Cyc. Pract. Med.*, Vol. iii, p. 44.—O'Brien,

Trans. Assoc. Phys. in Ireland, Vol. i, p. 54.—Begin, *Journ. Hebd. de Med. et Chir. Prat.*, 1830, Vol. i, p. 417.—Mouat, *Quart. Journ. of Med. and Phys. Soc. of Calcutta*, No. iii, July, 1837, (13 cases in which pus from the liver was apparently thrown off in a vicarious manner.)—Arnott, *Med. Chir. Trans.*, Vol. xv, (on the connection between injuries of the head and hepatic abscess.)—Dance, *Archiv. Generales*, t. xix, p. 172.—Cruveilhier, *Anat. Patholog. du Corps Humain*, Lib. ix, and *Dict. de Med. Prat.*, t. viii.—Bright, *Guy's Hosp. Reports*, Vol. v, and *Reports of Medical Cases*, 1827–31.—Conwell, *On the Liver*, 1835, p. 489, *seq.*—Bell, *On Diseases of the Liver*, Edin., 1833, p. 47.—Geddes, *Trans. of Med. and Phys. Soc. of Calcutta*, Vol. vi, p. 284, and *On Diseases of India*, Lond., 1846, p. 304.—Annesley, *On Diseases of India*, 4to, 1828, Vol. i, Sect. iii, p. 516, (splendid plates.)—Twining, *Diseases of Bengal, 2d Ed.*, Vol. i, p. 291.—Boyle, *Diseases of the Coast of Africa*, 1831, p. 365, (in one case abscess opened.)—Hawkins, *Med. Chir. Trans.*, xviii, p. 167, (cases of sloughing abscess.)—W. Thompson, *On Diseases of the Liver*, 8vo, 1841, pp. 32, 226, (contains much valuable information.)—Allan Webb, *Pathologia Indica, 2d Ed.*, 1848, p. 253, *seq.*—Parkes, *On Dysentery and Hepatitis in India*, Lond., 1846.—Budd, *On Diseases of the Liver*, 1*st Ed.*, p. 48.—Hare, *Med. Times*, July, 1852, p. 76.—*Med. Times*, Aug. 1852, p. 167.—Pavey, *ibid*, Jan. 1852, p. 15.—Dr. A. T. Thomson, *Lancet*, Vol. ii, 1847, p. 68, (opening into the lungs.)—*Lancet*, 1846, Vol. i, p. 302.—Sankey, *Lancet*, 1847, Vol. i, p. 286.—Parkes, *Lancet*, 1847, Vol. i, p. 336.—Norris, *Lancet*, Vol. ii, 1846, p. 375, (abscess opened—recovery.)—W. Smith, *Lancet*, 1846, Vol. ii, p. 497.—R. Thompson, *Lancet*, 1849, Vol. i, p. 232.—Dr. C. J. B. Williams, *Med. Gazette*, Vol. i, N. S., p. 1404, (curious case, abscess containing air, &c.)—Alexander, *Med. Gazette*, p. 1456.—Chambers, *Med. Gazette*, Vol. iii, p. 36.—Ross, *Med. Gazette*, Vol. v, p. 190.—H. Davies, *Med. Gazette*, Vol. vi, p. 908.—Sankey, *Med. Gazette*, Vol. iv, p. 516, (with pelvic abscess.)—Fuller, *Med. Gazette*, Vol. iv, p. 581, (abscess opening at umbilicus.)—Everett, *Med. Gazette*, Vol. iv, p. 949, (a very interesting case.)—R. W. Smith, *Dublin Med. Journal*, Vol. i, p. 247.—Hutton, *Dublin Med. Journal*, Sept. 1st, 1840, (abscess opened—death.)—Woodroofe, *Dub. Qu. Journal of Med. Sciences*, Vol. vi, 1848, p. 177.—Banks, *ibid*, Vol. xii, 1851, pp. 194, 199, (two cases.)—Harvey, *ibid*, Vol. x, p. 199.—Inman, *Edin. Med. Surg. Journal*, No. clx, p. 140.—Bentley, *Med. Gazette*, Dec. 22d, 1848, and *Ranking's Abstract*, Vol. ix, p. 249, (opening into the pericardium.)—Allan, *Lancet*, Vol. i, N. S., p. 644, (opening into the pericardium.)—Pierquin, *Journ. de Prog. des Sciences Med.*, t. xiv, p. 252.—Walshe, *Lancet*, 1849, Vol. ii, p. 525, (a very valuable Clinical Lecture, especially with reference to the urine in these cases.)—Raiken, *Lancet*, 1847, Vol. ii, p. 311, (on Abscesses opening into the lungs.)—Broussais, *Journ. de Med.*, Aug. and Sept. 1845, (Obs. in Algeria.)—Andral, *Clin. Medicale, 2d Ed.*, Vol. iv, p. 171.—

Schut of Vienna, *Wiener Zeitschrift*, Feb. 1846, *Ranking's Abstract*, iv, p. 60.—Henoch, *Klinik der Unterleibs-Krankheitan*, Berlin, 1852, and *Brit. and For. Med. Chir. Review*, July, 1854, p. 172.—Maclean, *Indian Annals of Medicine*, No. 3, p. 1, (on Mercury in Hepatic Affections.)—Several articles in the six volumes of the *Madras Med. Quart. Journal*, and in the *Trans. of the Med. and Phys. Societies of Bombay and Calcutta*.

APPENDIX.

Abscesses co-existing with the abscess in the liver were found in 9 cases—in the brain twice, (74, 240,) in the abdominal cavity twice, (16, 77,) and once in each of the following positions: perinæum, (234,) in one of the mesenteric glands, (237,) under the chin, (227,) in the lungs, (226,) and in various parts of the body, (244.) In two instances there were ulcers on the extremities at the time of admission, one on the elbow, (229,) and one on the leg, (232.) In the above cases, no communication was found to exist between these abscesses and that in the liver.

Nos. of peculiar or interesting cases. Abscess in the liver simulating abdominal aneurism, 228, 232—*simulating ventral hernia,* 234—*followed by abscess of the brain,* 240—*terminating in erysipelas simulating phlegmasia dolens,* 274—*proving fatal by hæmorrhage into the abscess,* 47, 226, 258—*a needle found imbedded in the abscess,* 194—*gall-bladder distended, simulating hepatic abscess,* 229—*gall-bladder removed by gangrene,* 5.

Abscess-walls—condition of, (*p.* 129.) 5, 7, 31, 41, 42, 46, 47, 50, 64, 77, 80, 83, 85, 87, 88, 89, 90, 91, 93, 95, 101, 103, 104, 108, 115, 118, 119, 122, 128, 135, 137, 142, 144, 146, 148, 151, 155, 156, 157, 162, 163, 168, 214, 216, 218, 219, 220, 223, 224, 226, 233, 235, 240, 242, 249, 251, 287.

Abscesses which burst spontaneously, (*p.* 131.) *Into the lungs,* 7, 10, 39, 50, 58, 64, 68, 82, 85, 99, 102, 122, 125, 130, 142, 147, 164, 180, 181, 182, 183, 196, 209, 236, 267, 272, 288, 291. *Into the thoracic cavity,* 16, 30, 53, 60, 62, 65, 69, 70, 73, 106, 224, 227, 283, 286. *Into the abdominal cavity,* 35, 133, 134, 135, 145, 148, 161, 179, 194, 231, 232, 239, 262, 263, 290. *Into the large intestines,* 5, 67, 138, 177, 178, 230, 298.

Vomiting and nausea, (*p.* 152.) 1, 7, 17, 19, 26, 30, 35, 40, 41, 44, 47, 55, 60, 79, 80, 81, 87, 90, 92, 100, 103, 104, 105, 114, 115, 116, 119, 122, 126, 138, 140, 141, 146, 150, 151, 157, 162, 163, 165, 166, 177, 182, 184, 185, 186, 189, 190, 192, 194, 195,

197, 198, 199, 200, 201, 202, 203, 204, 205, 206, 208, 210, 211, 212, 217, 220, 228, 230, 231, 234, 238, 240, 241, 291. *Absent*, 70, 144, 159, 187, 188, 191, 193, 196, 207, 209.

Mercury, cases in which its action is noticed, (p. 199.) 3, 4, 5, 6, 9, 12, 15, 16, 19, 20, 23, 24, 25, 26, 27, 31, 33, 35, 39, 54, 62, 68, 69, 70, 78, 79, 87, 88, 91, 93, 94, 95, 97, 103, 113, 130, 132, 133, 136, 141, 146, 151, 156, 159, 161, 162, 163, 170, 171, 172, 176, 178, 180, 181, 182, 183, 217, 225, 242.

It was purposed originally to have inserted an Appendix of much greater length, giving in detail the numbers of all the cases necessary to substantiate the statements made in the Analysis and Remarks; but in dividing them into classes, as mentioned in the Preface, some of them were unfortunately displaced, and it was found impossible to re-arrange them without devoting more time to it, than my other duties would permit. The whole of the statements, however, are believed to be substantially correct.

E. J. W.